Cardiac
Pearls

Cardiac
Pearls

W. Proctor Harvey, M.D.

Professor of Medicine
Division of Cardiology
•
Georgetown University
Medical Center
•
Washington, D.C.

Dedication

*To my beloved
daughter,
Janet Carolyn
Trivette, who
"grew up" to be the
young woman (wife
and mother) that her
mother, Irma and I
always hoped she
would.*

W. Proctor Harvey

About the Author

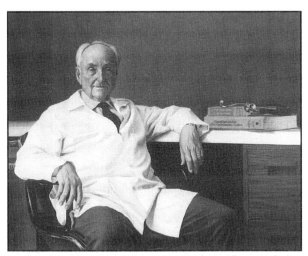

Portrait by Mary Ekroos, donated by Morris and Rose Kanfer.

W. Proctor Harvey, M.D. is Professor of Medicine at Georgetown University School of Medicine and former Director of the Division of Cardiology. He also serves or has served as a Consultant in Cardiology to the U.S. Department of State, Walter Reed Army Medical Center and Andrews Air Force Base Hospital in Washington, D.C., and to the U.S. Naval Hospital and the National Heart, Lung and Blood Institute.

Dr. Harvey has served as President of the American Heart Association and as President of the Association of University Cardiologists. He is a Master of the American College of Physicians, a Fellow of the American College of Cardiology and a Fellow of the Council of Clinical Cardiology of the American Heart Association.

Dr. Harvey is the co-author, with Samuel A. Levine, of the textbook, *Clinical Auscultation of the Heart,* former Editor-in-Chief of the monthly journals, *Current Problems in Cardiology,* and *Medical Times,* and a former Co-Editor of the Year Book Series, *Cardiology.*

Among the many honors Dr. Harvey has received are:

- Gifted Teacher Award, American College of Cardiology
- Distinguished Teacher Award, American College of Physicians
- Distinguished Service Award, World Congress of Cardiology
- James B. Herrick Award, given by the Council of Clinical Cardiology of the American Heart Association
- Gold Heart Award of the American Heart Association
- Patrick Healy Award and Honorary Degree of Doctor of Science of Georgetown University
- Honorary Degree of Doctor of Law and the Thomas Gibson Hobbs Memorial Award of Lynchburg College
- Helen Taussig Award, American Heart Association (Maryland Affiliate)
- 1978 Medalist, presented by the American College of Chest Physicians
- Distinguished Physicians Award (awarded by *Modern Medicine)*
- Ray C. Fish Award of the Texas Heart Institute
- Laureate Award, American College of Physicians
- Alpha Omega Alpha, the national medical honor society, Distinguished Teacher Award (given in conjunction with the Association of American Medical Colleges). Stated in the citation: "Dr. Harvey is known worldwide for his teaching skills, for his contributions of innovative teaching and to medical education and for his exemplary dedication to medicine and his patients."

Dr. Harvey is a graduate of Duke University School of Medicine and was a recipient of its Distinguished Alumnus Award. He trained at Peter Bent Brigham Hospital, Boston, and served on the staff there, before joining the faculty of Georgetown University School of Medicine in 1950.

Contents

Preface

This book is not like other textbooks of medicine and cardiology. In fact, most of these cardiac pearls will not be found in today's textbooks. They represent a compilation of valuable clinical observations over a number of decades. They have stood the test of time and focus on the *patient* who, unfortunately, at present is too often relegated to the "back burner."

Cardiac Pearls is purposely designed so that you can open it and begin reading at any point, encompassing as many pearls as you can cover in the time you have available. The table of contents allows you to select those pearls relating to a specific aspect of cardiovascular disease. Each pearl is set in bold face type and is preceded by a pearl-shaped black dot ●.

Introduction

We tend to forget that the great majority of diagnoses of cardiovascular disease can be and are made in the office or at the bedside. Usually, we do not need the sophisticated, elegant laboratory diagnostic equipment that we all have in our modern hospitals. The diagnosis can be accomplished by combining the findings of a complete cardiovascular evaluation — a careful, detailed history and physical examination, electrocardiogram, x-ray, and simple laboratory tests. This is known as the "five finger" method of diagnosis. Making a fist provides a powerful, effective and accurate clinical diagnosis.

The history (thumb) is generally the most important finger; next is the physical exam (index finger). Often, by the time these two have been completed, the diagnosis is already evident. Too often, today, these simple basic important components of evaluation of a patient are neglected or deemphasized. Specialized "invasive" or "non invasive" laboratory procedures are often top priority, which may be unnecessary, expensive and sometimes even risky.

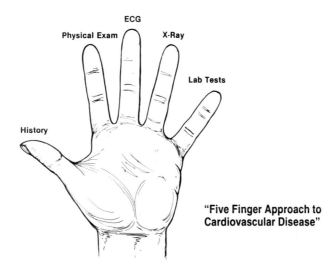

"Five Finger Approach to Cardiovascular Disease"

Pulsus Alternans, Alternation of Heart Sounds and Murmurs, and Ventricular Gallops

● **On Greeting the Patient — Valuable information is often obtained by greeting and shaking hands with our patient, and then moving our index and middle fingers over the hand to palpate the radial artery (Figure 1).**

Most physicians do not do this, and thereby are missing a unique opportunity to know that the patient has heart disease.

Palpating the pulse may indicate that it alternates in amplitude with each beat: strong, weak, strong, weak. This is pulsus alternans (Figure 2), which is nothing new; in fact, Sir Thomas Lewis described this many years ago, in his textbook, "The Mechanism and Graphic Registration of the Heart Beat." Every other beat is weaker than the preceding one, and after a premature beat, the alternation is more accentuated.

● **We will not detect the pulsus alternans if we palpate with very firm pressure over the artery; instead, we need to use very light pressure, similar to what might be felt by a blow of breath on our fingers.**

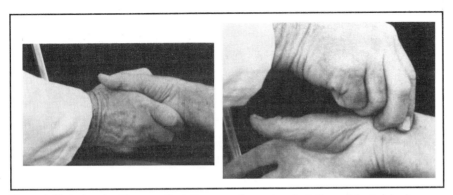

Figure 1: Shake hands with your patient; then move fingers to palpate the radial arterial pulse. Valuable information may be obtained from this simple, infrequently used maneuver.

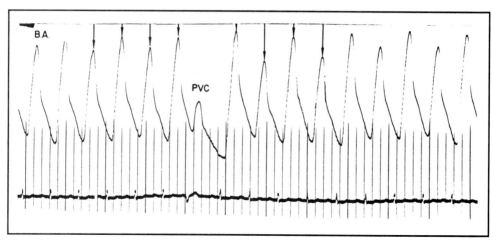

Figure 2: Pulsus Alternans — Note alternation of the brachial arterial pulse (B.A.) is accentuated following a premature ventricular contraction (PVC).

Pulsus alternans is a common finding, but we have to look for it. As is true in all of medicine — we find what we look for. However, there are two parts to this observation. Not only do we find what we look for, but we have to *know* what we are looking for; then we will find it.

- **When we find the pulsus alternans, if we then search carefully on auscultation, we will hear alternation of the second heart sound in the great majority of patients (Figure 3).**

The first sound can also alternate in intensity, although it may not be as easily detected as the second sound. If a murmur is present, it too will alternate in intensity. A ventricular (S_3) diastolic gallop also should be heard (Figure 4), provided simple, basic techniques, to be discussed, are used.

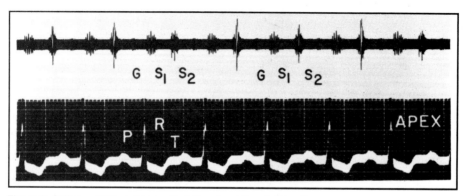

Figure 3: Gallop — Note ventricular diastolic gallop (G) and alternation of the second heart sound (S_2).

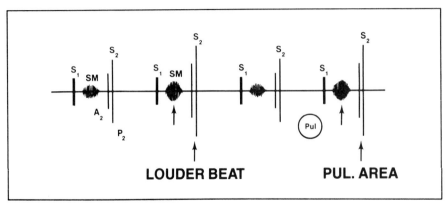

Figure 4: Alternation of Intensity — Note alternation of intensity of both second sound (S₂) and systolic murmur (SM) every other beat.

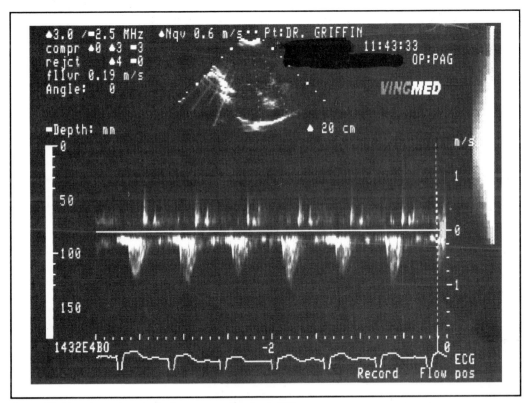

Figure 4A: Note alternation of velocity on every other beat of this Doppler echocardiogram. This correlates with pulsus alternans and alternation of the systolic murmur heard with the stethoscope.
Courtesy Dr. John Griffin, Springfield, Mass.

Thus, it often takes less than several minutes to know that our patient has heart disease. These findings, which can be detected in the examiner's office or at the bedside, establish the clinical diagnosis of cardiac decompensation.

As a rule, the more prominent these findings, and the more easily found, the greater the degree of heart failure. Pulsus alternans can be one of its most subtle signs, but we must look for it. We must then specifically search for the ventricular (S_3) gallop, and alternation of the sounds and murmurs. A method personally used:

- **Carefully *inspect* the patient's body lying supine (Figure 5A).**

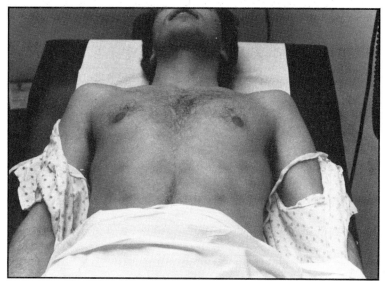

Figure 5A: Inspection should be part of every physical exam. Take time to *look* carefully.

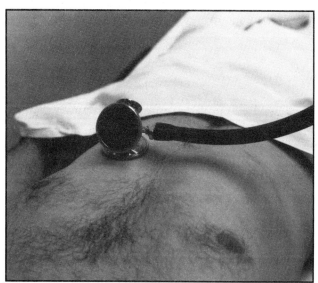

Figure 5B: Lower Left Sternal Border — The stethoscope is placed along the lower left sternal border, providing an overview for auscultation of heart sounds and murmurs.

- **Then place the stethoscope along the patient's lower left sternal border, thereby providing an overview (Figure 5B): Listen specifically to the first sound; then the second sound; then systematically listen for sounds in systole, murmurs in systole, sounds in diastole, and murmurs in diastole.**

In this way we are dissecting, so to speak, the various heart sounds and murmurs of the heart cycle. We are not trying to listen to everything at once. This is analogous to listening to the music played by a symphony orchestra. One is able to pick out a particular instrument such as a violin, horn, flute, piano, or kettle drum, if we concentrate on it.

After detecting a pulsus alternans, focus on listening for a sound occurring in early to mid-diastole. A faint third heart sound is present, which has the timing of a ventricular (S_3) gallop. A simple but important cardiac pearl:

- **Turn the patient to the left lateral position and palpate with the index and middle fingers of the left hand to locate the point of maximum impulse of the left ventricle. Hold that spot with the fingers, and place the bell of the stethoscope lightly over this localized area (Figure 6); the ventricular (S_3) gallop may now be louder and more clearly heard.**

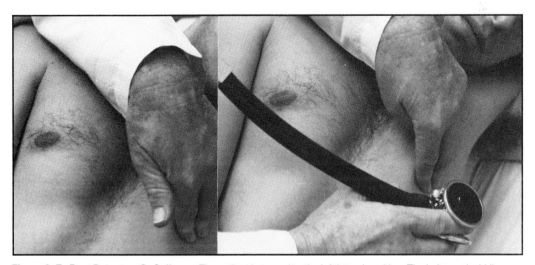

Figure 6: To Best Detect an S_3 Gallop — The patient is turned to the left lateral position. The index and middle fingers of the left hand palpate the point of maximal impulse of the left ventricle; holding that spot, the bell of the stethoscope is placed lightly over it, barely making an air seal with the skin of the chest wall.

The gallop may also alternate in intensity with every other beat. Pressure on the stethoscope can eliminate this gallop.

We now have noted in this patient: pulsus alternans of the radial pulse observed when first greeting our patient, alternation of the first and second sounds, and systolic murmur and ventricular (S₃) gallop, also alternating in intensity. With these clinical cardiac pearls, we have definitely diagnosed cardiac decompensation. This has been promptly accomplished in the office, or at the bedside, and without having to utilize expensive procedures. Too few physicians utilize this information, first obtained as a pearl by feeling the radial pulse.

Occasionally a colleague may say, "Why do you talk about the radial pulse, when the brachial, carotid, and femoral pulses are larger arteries, and more easily palpated?"

The answer is that of course we use these other arteries to obtain valuable information; but after greeting our patient for the first time, it is easy and natural to move the palpating fingers gently to the radial pulse, which quickly provides information and is often reassuring to the apprehensive and nervous patient with the 'laying on of the hands'. Although all pulses are subsequently examined, one does not immediately palpate the carotid and even less likely the femoral artery.

- **Another cardiac pearl: A faint gallop, ventricular (S₃), and or atrial (S₄) might be overlooked in a patient having an emphysematous chest with an increase in AP diameter due to chronic obstructive pulmonary disease. This is true if one listens over the usual areas of the precordium, the lower left sternal border and apex; however, by listening over the xiphoid area or epigastric area, it might be easily detected (Figures 7, 8, and 9).**

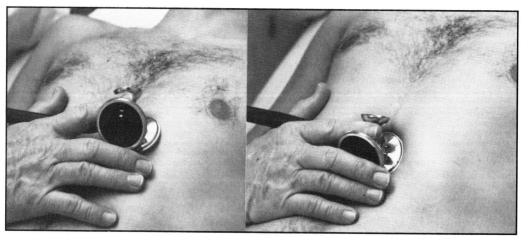

Figure 7: Importance of Listening over the Xiphoid and Epigastric Areas — Left: Heart sounds and murmurs can be faint and poorly heard over the usual areas of the precordium of an emphysematous chest, but are clearly heard by listening over the xiphoid and epigastrium (right).

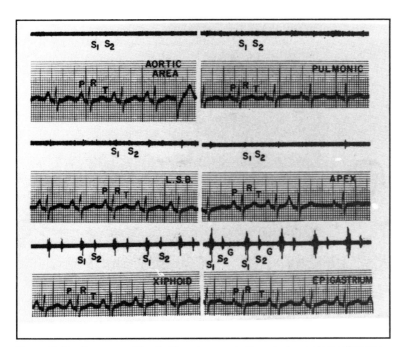

Figure 8: Emphysema — Chest with an increase in the anterior-posterior diameter due to emphysema from chronic obstructive pulmonary disease. The heart sounds can be faint (top and middle tracings) and difficult to hear. Gallops might not be detected over the lower left sternal border (L.S.B.) and apex; however, by listening over the xiphoid process (lower tracing), and/or epigastric area, the heart sounds (S_1, S_2) and gallop (G) are heard.

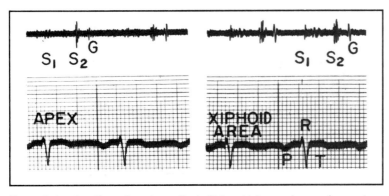

Figure 9: Another Example — In a patient with heart failure and an emphysematous chest, heart sounds (S_1, S_2) and a faint gallop (G) might be better heard over the xiphoid area than over the apex.

With advanced degrees of cardiac decompensation (the ejection fraction is low), these physical signs, as might be expected, are more easily detected; they become more difficult to find as improvement takes place (the ejection fraction is higher). If they are no longer present, the decompensation has been eliminated (the ejection fraction is now likely in normal range). The ejection fraction determined in the diagnostic laboratory is a way of determining the degree of cardiac decompensation. At times, it is a very helpful test; however it can be used too frequently, and adds expense to the patient and might be spared if the physician pays attention to these clinical findings.

Gallops

- **Best Position to Hear Gallops** — The diastolic filling sounds, S_3 and S_4, at times may be heard only when the patient is turned to the left lateral position and one listens over the point of maximal impulse with the bell of the stethoscope barely making a seal with the skin of the chest wall (Figures 10, 11, and 12).

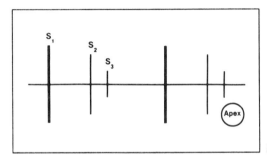

Figure 10: Ventricular Diastolic Gallop (S_3).

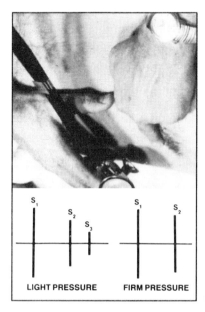

Figure 11: Light and Firm Pressure — With the patient turned to the left lateral position apply light pressure with the bell of the stethoscope; a ventricular gallop (S_3) is easily heard. Firm pressure diminishes or eliminates the third sound.

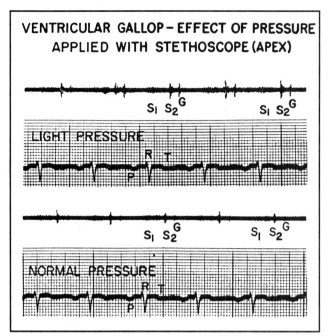

VENTRICULAR GALLOP — EFFECT OF PRESSURE APPLIED WITH STETHOSCOPE (APEX)

Figure 12: Another Example of Pressure — Use light pressure with the bell of the stethoscope to better detect a faint ventricular gallop (G).

Pressure on the stethoscope can eliminate these sounds. Alternating the pressure causes the sounds to be "in" or "out," thereby positively identifying them. Listen immediately after the patient turns, since these sounds (particularly the normal physiological S_3 and the S_3 ventricular gallop) may be transient.

Remember, this position and the point of maximal impulse also is the best way to detect the diastolic rumble of mitral stenosis.

Sometimes, if searched for, both S_3 and S_4 gallops can be heard over the supraclavicular area of the neck.

A question frequently asked is how to tell the difference between an S_4, a split first sound, and an ejection sound? Listening at the lower left sternal border or apex, as just described, the S_4 is eliminated with pressure on the stethoscope. Pressure does not eliminate the ejection sound nor the splitting of the S_1. The S_4 is usually not heard over the aortic area, whereas the aortic ejection sound *is* so detected. The mitral and tricuspid components of the normal split of the first sound are closer and sound alike, and over the aortic area only one component of S_1 is generally heard.

- **An atrial gallop (S_4) is frequently found in patients having coronary heart disease. It should be specifically searched for in all patients with coronary heart disease.**

For example, in a patient who has a history of a myocardial infarction in the past, an S_4 is an expected finding (Figure 13). If it isn't found, one might wonder if such a diagnosis was correct.

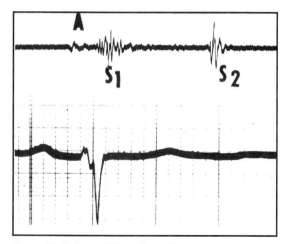

Figure 13: Gallop — This patient with coronary artery disease has an atrial gallop (A) heard while listening at the apex.

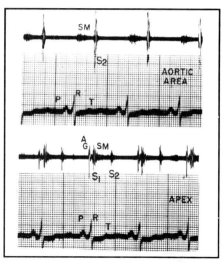

Figure 14: Hypertensive Gallop — Atrial (S₄) gallop (AG) heard at apex — not over aortic area. Note prominent "tambour" second sound (S₂) and systolic murmur (SM) at aortic area. The usual atrial (S₄) gallop is fainter than was heard in this patient.

- **The S₄ is a constant finding in patients who have hypertension. It does not denote cardiac decompensation, as does the S₃ (ventricular gallop) with its accompanying pulsus alternans, alternation of the second sound, and alternation of murmurs.**

A hypertensive patient may have an S₄ heard for as long as 10 or 15 years or longer and without cardiac decompensation; however, once heart failure occurs, the ventricular (S₃) gallop will occur.

In a patient with mild to severe hypertension, in addition to the S₄, a "tambour" second sound is heard, particularly with higher levels of blood pressure. In years past, the tambour second sound was a sign of luetic aortitis. However, today its most common cause is hypertension. Another auscultatory finding with hypertension is a short early to mid systolic murmur over the aortic area and sometimes also at the apex (Figure 14).

Physicians differ as to when to start antihypertensive therapy in a patient having milder degrees of blood pressure elevation. Some give medication if the blood pressure is 160/100, others 150/96, 158/104, 160/110, and so forth. A personal approach is that, if a patient has an atrial (S₄) sound in presystole alone, and the blood pressure is constantly around 140/90 or above, medication is indicated. The presence of an S₄ indicates that the heart has already been affected. If a tambour S₂ and an aortic systolic murmur is present, it would be further justification for treatment.

The atrial (S₄) diastolic gallop also can be present in a patient having only a prolongation of the P-R interval on the electrocardiogram.

- **Ventricular Diastolic Gallop** — As a rule, a ventricular (S₃) diastolic gallop is not a loud sound. In fact, most gallops are faint and one needs to listen very carefully and specifically for them. They are very common, however. Most ventricular (S₃) gallops are usually heard every third or fourth beat rather than with every beat. On the other hand, an atrial (S₄) gallop is more likely to be heard with almost every beat.

As previously mentioned, faint gallop sounds (S₃ and S₄) can often be detected by listening with the bell of the stethoscope placed lightly over the lower left sternal border.

- **Ventricular Gallop After Tachycardia** — A ventricular (S₃) diastolic gallop may be temporarily heard after a prolonged period of rapid tachycardia such as paroxysmal atrial tachycardia in a person who has a normal heart. It is generally of no specific significance and does not connote heart disease. The gallop sound usually disappears after a period of minutes to hours. Such a gallop does not carry the same connotation as the ventricular gallop of heart failure that is present continuously.

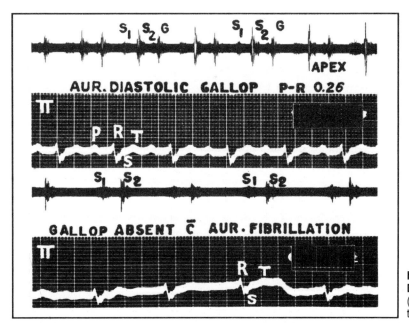

Figure 15: The Gallop Disappears — The atrial (S₄) gallop disappears with the onset of atrial fibrillation.

- An old teaching is that gallops disappear with atrial fibrillation. This is true of the atrial (S_4) (Figure 15) gallop (since there is no atrial contraction), but not of the ventricular (S_3) gallop, which persists.

Other Gallops

Occasionally, a physician will talk about a "Tennessee" gallop or a "Kentucky" gallop with the Ten-nes-see being an S_4 gallop and the Ken-tuck-y gallop an S_3 gallop. It is best to discontinue such descriptions because they can cause confusion. By use of the inching technique as described elsewhere, the correct identification of the type of gallop can be readily determined.

The question is sometimes asked, "What is the 'choo-choo train' murmur?" This is a term that has been applied to a murmur that resembles a train coming up an incline or out of a tunnel and it has been said to be specific for Ebstein's anomaly. However, the sounds and murmurs of Ebstein's do not remind me of the sounds coming from a "choo-choo train." It is best to simply describe the auscultatory events that occur.

Congestive Heart Failure

- **Early Signs:** The earliest physical signs of cardiac decompensation are not chest rales, jugular venous pulse distension, liver enlargement or peripheral edema. Rather, the finding of pulsus alternans and a ventricular (S_3) diastolic gallop can be the earliest, most subtle finding of cardiac decompensation.

Accompanying this, as discussed, may be alternation of the second sound, alternation of a murmur if present, and a ventricular (S_3) diastolic gallop.

- **Hydrothorax can be a complication of advanced congestive heart failure.**

It is not seen as frequently now as it was in the past — due to better present day medical treatment. Hydrothorax accompanying heart failure may be bilateral, but in my experience is more commonly present in the right thorax. This is probably best explained by simple gravity and the fact that these patients are more likely to lie and sleep on their right side rather than their left. Patients having enlarged hearts, often with an arrhythmia, such as atrial fibrillation, are conscious of their heart action when lying on their left side; therefore most prefer to sleep on their right side, and/or back.

When a left hydrothorax is present in a patient with heart disease, rule out the possibility of an etiology other than heart failure. I recall such a patient who had tuberculosis.

- **Cheyne-Stokes Respiration — Cheyne-Stokes respiration as a manifestation of heart failure is generally missed, simply because it is not looked for.**

Remember, while we find what we look for, we also must *know* what we are looking for. If the patient is not under the influence of a sedative or a narcotic, and if there is no significant cerebrovascular disease present, the presence of Cheyne-Stokes respiration usually indicates the patient has very advanced heart failure.

Personally observed have been a number of patients who had not been considered to have heart failure and the Cheyne-Stokes respiration had not been noted. This finding alone should alert the physician to promptly institute all necessary measures and medications to alleviate the cardiac decompensation.

- **Cardiac Pearl: Adequate auscultation may be accomplished during the apneic phases of Cheyne-Stokes respiration, but may be impossible during the dyspneic phase.**

- **Change of Normal Sinus Rhythm to Atrial Fibrillation — A patient with heart disease may have no evidence of cardiac decompensation, but acute pulmonary edema can occur with the change from normal sinus rhythm to atrial fibrillation. In some patients, this also may be the first indication of underlying heart disease.**

I have personally observed a lady of about 60 years of age who was admitted to the Emergency Room of a hospital with acute pulmonary edema, which occurred following the onset of atrial fibrillation. She was given digitalis, but even in increasing doses it did not control her fibrillation. She was transferred to another hospital for evaluation. It was finally realized that, whereas most patients' atrial fibrillation can be slowed with digoxin, hers could not. Verapamil, however, was successful in converting the ventricular rate to normal, and with quinidine she reverted to normal sinus rhythm. However, after a few days, she changed back into atrial fibrillation. She was again reverted to normal sinus rhythm, but maintenance quinidine did not prevent her atrial fibrillation.

- **When it is not possible to control atrial fibrillation after trying several antiarrhythmic drugs, it may be best for both physician and patient to accept and live with a chronic atrial fibrillation with a ventricular rate in the 60s or 70s.**

Chronic Fatigue

"I go to bed tired. I get up tired." I have heard patients say this for many years. This is the chronic fatigue that is a prominent symptom of chronic heart failure. It is to be expected and often can be helped by a general "tightening" of the patient's medical management.

The basic treatment of congestive heart failure is as follows:
1. Dietary restriction of sodium
2. Diuretics
3. ACE inhibitors
4. Digitalis
5. Vasodilators
6. Control of arrhythmias, if possible
7. Restriction of unnecessary physical activities.
8. Search for "reversible" or "curable" causes of heart failure (cardiac surgery, pulmonary emboli, infections, drug toxicity)
9. Patient education

Diuretics are a fundamental mainstay in treating heart failure. Chlorothiazide, introduced several decades ago, represented a major breakthrough in inducing diuresis of edema fluid; diazide diuretics (Diuril, Hydrodiuril) remain important drugs in treatment. We now have many effective diuretic agents that vary in potency.

For the patient having a mild to moderate degree of cardiac decompensation, the very potent diuretics such as furosemide (Lasix), ethacrynic acid (Edecrin), and butemetanide (Bumex) are not necessary. Instead, chlorothiazide or hydrochlorothiazide are usually satisfactory and less likely to be associated with complications such as electrolyte imbalance.

The intermittent use of diuretics is effective for mild to moderate decompensation. Some patients need a diuretic only once or twice a week rather than daily. For some women, I have suggested they take a tablet only once a month when they have their premenstrual edema.

- **Diuretics may be more effective on the days when there is less physical activity and more rest takes place.**

I have seen many patients who have little or no diuretic response during the busy weekdays, but on a quiet restful Sunday have a prompt significant response to their diuretic tablet of that day.

Of course, with more *advanced degrees of heart failure,* the stronger diuretics are needed and necessary. Combinations of diuretics, two or even three, can be effective in these patients whereas only one is not.

Hypokalemia (potassium depletion) may be a complication of diuretic therapy. In addition to loss of sodium in the urine, potassium also may be excreted to such a degree that hypokalemia results. Symptoms of fatigue, weakness and general malaise are clues to suspect this side effect of diuretic therapy and to prevent and treat with supplemental potassium (usually potassium chloride). Serum potassium levels should be checked at intervals to maintain the proper normal level.

It is important to remember that, while many hypokalemic patients complain of weakness and fatigue, others will be asymptomatic. Also, remember that potassium loss can occur with diarrhea and the excessive use of laxatives.

Patients should be advised to eat more of the foods having a higher potassium content. These are:

Very Good Sources of Potassium

Avocadoes
Bananas
Cantaloupe
Dandelions
Dates
Garlic
Kohlrabi
Lima beans
Melon, honeydew
Nectarine
Parsley
Parsnips
Potatoes
Swiss chard

Good Sources of Potassium

Artichokes
Beets
Beet greens
Blackberries
Broccoli
Brussel sprouts
Celeriac
Collards
Cucumbers
Greens
Kale
Mushrooms
Oranges
Orange juice
Peaches
Plantains
Pumpkins
Prunes
Prune juice
Rutabaga
Spinach
Strawberries
Sweet potatoes
Tomatoes
Tomato juice
Watermelon
Winter squash

Fair Sources of Potassium

Apples
Apricots
Asparagus
Beans, snap
Blueberries
Cabbage
Carrots
Cauliflower
Celery
Cherries
Corn
Cranberries
Eggplant
Grapefruit
Grapefruit juice
Grapes
Lemons
Lettuce
Limes
Mangos
Okra
Papayas
Peppers (green)
Pineapple
Pineapple juice
Plums
Pomegranates
Radishes
Raspberries
Rhubarb

Salsify
Shallots
Sprouts
Squash
Tangerine
Turnips
Watercress

Source: American Heart Association

Ideally, supply a list for the patient to keep and refer to. A word of caution: In patients with coronary artery disease who have already had a myocardial infarction and are taking digitalis and diuretics, low serum potassium can precipitate ventricular arrhythmias, including tachycardia, fibrillation, and death. Monitoring the serum potassium at intervals is a precautionary measure. Also, this should be done with elderly patients and alcoholics, because poor nutrition (poor appetite and decreased food intake) depletes potassium; also, they may be taking diuretics.

Dietary restriction of sodium. This is one of the most important aspects of treatment; it is also one of the most neglected.

Think how often we see patients with heart disease and failure who are taking an appropriate drug or drugs but do not restrict the sodium intake in their diet. Too often the patient is allowed to eat what he or she wants, thinking that a good diuretic will take care of it. It is particularly important for patients having more advanced degrees of cardiac decompensation to restrict their sodium intake. I still find this to be the most common need for "tightening" and improving their symptoms. Many patients are told to "cut down on the salt" but no specific dietary education and counseling is given. Many patients say that they are on sodium restriction, but questioning them about what they eat for each meal quickly identifies no significant restriction. In addition, when discussing diet with some of our clinic patients, they may be aware of the need to eat less salty foods, but unfortunately, because of their low income, they have to eat more of the higher sodium content foods such as processed meats and canned soup; however, these patients can still be advised which foods in particular to avoid.

Sodium restriction is number one in treatment of more advanced degrees of cardiac decompensation. Despite the use of drugs, benefit to the patient may not occur unless there is rigid sodium restriction.

Of course, with mild cardiac decompensation, more moderate restriction of salt in the diet may suffice (not adding extra salt to food when eating, or only adding a small amount to make it "tasty").

A cardiac pearl to know that a patient is adhering to his low sodium diet is when he says: "The food is too salty when I eat in restaurants or away from home". I have heard this unsolicited statement from many patients.

Also beneficial is to encourage our patients to become experts on low sodium diets and to learn and use "gourmet" low sodium food preparation. For example, using wine and herbs can make their food more palatable. Many books are available to every patient — in bookstores, libraries, and from heart associations.

Patients needing strict sodium restriction should be educated concerning their diet by the physician and/or nurse, dietician or medical assistant. Local American Heart Association chapters can aid in supplying information and diet lists for individual patients.

Salt substitutes are frequently used by patients adhering to a low salt diet. Potassium chloride is commonly a basic component of these substitutes. Having tested some of those myself, I found that a smaller amount of the substitute is required to simulate a "salt" taste than regular salt; if more is used, a bitter taste is produced. It is helpful for any medical personnel recommending salt substitutes to try them on their own.

Vinegar is a substitute that many have used and liked.

The following are *not* salt substitutes: Onion salt, celery salt, garlic salt. However, they may be confused with salt (sodium chloride) substitutes. You would think that everyone would know that these are regular salt combined with the other ingredients to add extra flavor to food. However, don't take it for granted and remind your patients that these do not represent real substitutes. Illustrating this confusion was a physicist who happily exclaimed "I don't mind the salt substitute at all; in fact I like it. I use celery salt."

Reduction of physical activity. Daily periods of rest, lying down, often with the legs elevated on pillows can be recommended if it is possible.

In some, taking a tub bath with the feet propped up has been helpful in mobilizing edema fluid in the legs. The tub should be well filled with water. The patient having cardiac decompensation does not need a strenuous exercise program such as jogging, stationary bike, weights and "jazzercise." In fact, these activities may be detrimental.

Concerning advice to a patient about physical activity, remember the old fashioned rule: Do what you do in comfort, avoiding extremes of exertion in extremes of weather (the bitter cold is the worst, and the hot humid is the next).

● **A headache drug that may possibly produce heart disease is Sansert (methysergide maleate).**

Fibrotic thickening of heart valves can occur. I have personally observed several patients whose aortic regurgitation seemed to be related to the use of this drug. Also, I remember a patient whose myocardial infarction might have been related to coronary artery fibrosis producing occlusion. Retroperitoneal fibrosis and pleuro-pulmonary fibrosis have also been reported.

The drug is apparently useful for management of severe headache; physicians prescribing this medicine should be aware of the possible complications.

Inching Technique

- **The inching technique is the most accurate and practical way of timing extra heart sounds and murmurs.**

  The stethoscope is moved or "inched" downward over the precordium from the aortic area to the apex. You can also start at the apex and lower left sternal border and inch upward towards the base of the heart. Both directions should be utilized. If an extra sound is present and needs to be identified as being systolic or diastolic the inching technique can immediately and accurately identify it.

- **First, start over the aortic area, remembering that the second heart sound over the aortic area is almost always louder than the first (Figure 16).**

  The second sound may not be loud, but of normal intensity. However, it is louder than the first sound over this area. The second sound, of course, signals the end of systole.

  By keeping the second sound in mind and using it as a reference, move the stethoscope by progressively inching from the aortic area down to the apex (Figure 17). If the extra sound is in systole, it occurs before the second heart sound at the lower left sternal border and apex and is therefore a systolic sound, such as a systolic click. The systolic click is generally not heard over the aortic area.

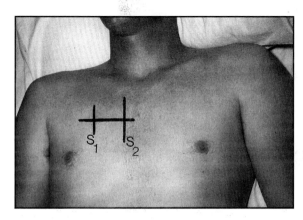

Figure 16: Intensity: Normally, the second sound (S_2) over the aortic area is louder than the first sound (S_1).

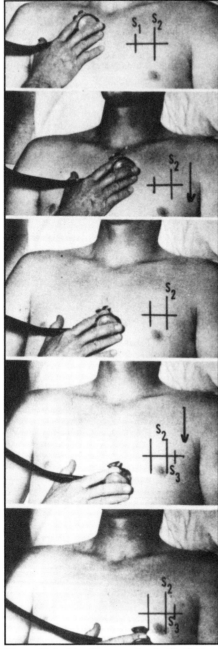

Figure 17: Inching Downward — Inching from the aortic area down to the apex. Note S₃ appears after the second sound (S₂) in the two lower panels.

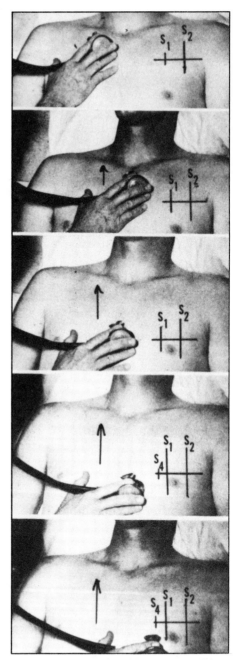

Figure 18: Inching upward from the lower left sternal border to the aortic area. Keeping the first sound (S₁) as reference, the S₄ is heard in presystole but disappears in the middle tracing and subsequent positions, including the aortic area.

Your stethoscope can now be inched upward and you will note that the extra sound disappears when you reach the aortic area.

A sound in diastole can be detected by inching down from the aortic area; using the second heart sound as a reference, the sound, when listening along the lower left sternal border, now is heard coming shortly after the second sound; it is therefore a diastolic sound such as a ventricular (S_3) gallop or a normal third heart sound.

When you reverse the inching and move from the apex and lower left sternal border, the sound in early diastole disappears as the stethoscope is inched up to the base of the heart (Figure 18). If there is an extra sound occurring just before the first heart sound, the inching should start at the lower left sternal border and then the stethoscope is gradually inched up to the aortic area. A sound occurring just before the first heart sound is heard along the lower left sternal border and apex. Now, keeping the *first heart sound* in mind as a reference, the extra sound will disappear at about the third left sternal border, and will not be heard over the aortic area. This is typical of the atrial (S_4) gallop.

- **Commonly, two diastolic gallops are present in the patient having cardiac decompensation associated with dilated cardiomyopathy, coronary artery disease, or hypertensive heart disease (Figures 19 and 20).**

One readily hears gallop rhythm with the stethoscope, but frequently it is assumed that only one gallop is heard, whereas in fact, both atrial (S_4) and ventricular (S_3) gallops are present. To detect both, first inch from the aortic area to the apex, keeping the second heart sound in mind. When the stethoscope reaches the lower left sternal border and apex, the extra sound is identified as coming in early diastole and is, therefore, a ventricular (S_3) gallop.

Now inch upward from the lower left sternal border to the aortic area, keeping the first heart sound in mind as a reference; an extra sound present in presystole now disappears along the third left sternal border and is still not heard up to the aortic

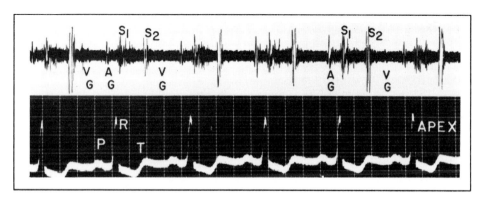

Figure 19: Two Gallops — This patient has hypertension, coronary artery disease, and congestive heart failure. Note both atrial (A_G) and ventricular (V_G) diastolic gallops.

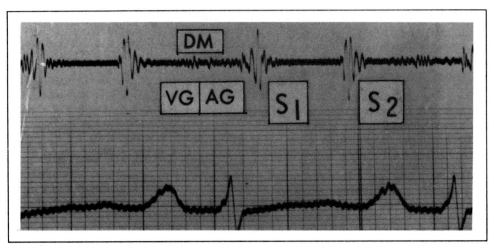

Figure 20: Rumble — A patient with both atrial (AG) and ventricular (VG) diastolic gallops. Note the two gallops are in close proximity, producing a short diastolic rumble murmur (DM). A reminder that "all that rumbles is not mitral stenosis."

area. This is the atrial (S_4) gallop. The inching upwards and downwards can be repeated, and by utilizing the inching technique, one can accurately identify the presence of both gallop sounds.

When these two diastolic sounds occur in close proximity (both having low frequency after-vibrations) a short rumbling diastolic murmur may be heard. In fact, in the past, we had two patients referred for mitral commissurotomy because of the presence of a diastolic rumble. An erroneous diagnosis of mitral stenosis had been made because the gallop sounds occurred in close proximity as diastole shortened with an increase in heart rate. With a still faster heart rate, which further shortens diastole, the two sounds can, on rare occasions, occur at *exactly* the same time. This is a *summation* gallop (Figure 21), which can be loud — even louder than the first or second sound and therefore misinterpreted as either the first or second sound. This mistake, however, should not occur if the cardiac pearl of inching is employed.

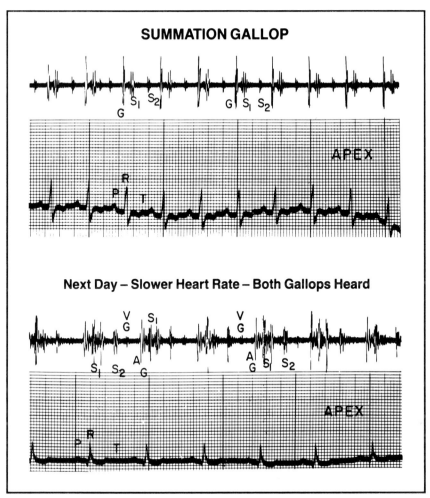

Figure 21: Summation gallop (top) (G) in a patient with hypertensive heart disease and congestive failure. Bottom: Next day. Loud summation gallop absent, atrial (A_G) and ventricular (V_G) gallops now readily identified.

Aortic Regurgitation

- **Positions and Techniques for Auscultation** — The murmurs of aortic regurgitation (including the faintest) are generally best heard when the patient is sitting upright, leaning forward, breath held in deep expiration; use firm pressure of the flat diaphragm of the stethoscope and listen along the third left sternal border (Figure 22).

- **Firm pressure on the stethoscope** — enough to leave an imprint of the diaphragm chest piece on the chest wall (Figure 22) — may be necessary to bring out a faint murmur of grade 1 or 2 intensity.

I always tell my patient that I will press firmly on the stethoscope. "You will feel this, but it should not cause discomfort. Let me know if it does." No discomfort to the patient results, as a rule. Also, alerting the patient to expect the pressure of the stethoscope is obviously beneficial in performing this maneuver.

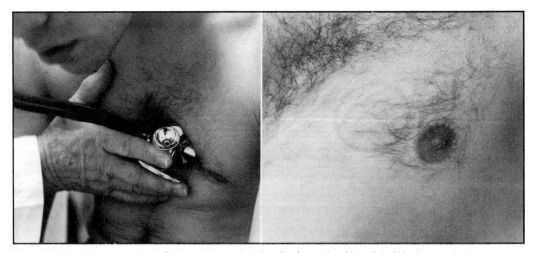

Figure 22: Firm Pressure — Left: Patient sitting upright, leaning forward and breath held in deep expiration; listening with the flat diaphragm and exerting firm pressure against the chest wall. Right: Enough pressure was exerted to leave a momentary imprint of the chest piece on the skin of the chest.

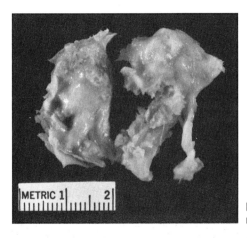

Figure 23: Pathology — Acute aortic regurgitation due to infective endocarditis.

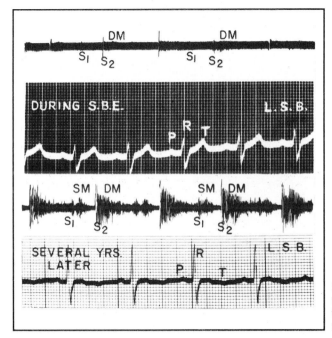

Figure 24: Infective endocarditis (SBE) changes a minimal leak of the aortic valve to a severe one requiring surgical replacement of the aortic valve.

Use this pearl when examining all of your patients — it may help you to detect a faint murmur from a minimal aortic valve lesion. Such a murmur could be a first clue, along with an ejection sound, of a congenital bicuspid aortic valve.

I have frequently said, "Please don't overlook a faint aortic diastolic murmur. If you are going to overlook a murmur, it would be better to miss a loud one, since such a murmur would obviously be detected by others." If a faint grade 1 or 2 aortic diastolic murmur, as may occur with a bicuspid aortic valve, is overlooked, the patient can have serious complications such as infective endocarditis, which can damage the aortic valve to a degree that significant, advanced aortic regurgitation results, necessitating aortic valve replacement (Figures 23 and 24).

Antibiotic prophylaxis against infective endocarditis as outlined by the American Heart Association should be given for dental procedures (including cleaning and filling of teeth as well as extractions), as well as certain surgical, gastrointestinal and genitourinary procedures. See p. 83.

- **A faint aortic diastolic murmur might be overlooked if only the bell chest piece of the stethoscope is used. The flat diaphragm is necessary and should be used to examine all patients.**

Poorly appreciated and seldom used are other positions for auscultation of a diastolic murmur of aortic regurgitation:
1. The patient lying on his or her stomach (prone) and propped up on the elbows (Figure 25). This position is also especially useful to detect a pericardial friction rub which might be missed if it is not searched for with the patient in this position.
2. The patient standing, leaning forward with his or her hands against a wall (Figure 26). A quiet room should always be used, if possible.

Right-sided Murmurs of Aortic Regurgitation — The great majority of murmurs of aortic regurgitation are heard louder at the *left* sternal border compared with the counterpart on the right (Figure 27). However, some aortic diastolic murmurs are best heard along the *right* sternal border rather than the *left* (Figure 28).

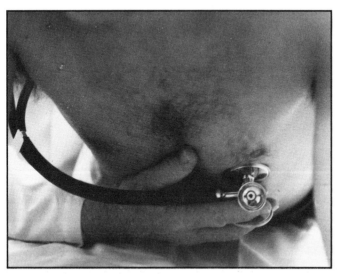

Figure 25: Patient lying on his stomach propped up on his elbows.
Firm pressure is applied, using the flat diaphragm of the stethoscope. The aortic diastolic murmur will usually be best heard over the third left sternal border. A pericardial friction rub can often be detected in this position, as would a decrease in intensity of heart sounds and murmurs in some patients having pericardial effusion.

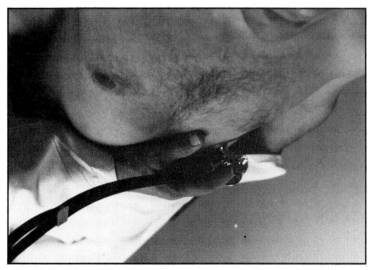

Figure 26: Listening for a Faint Murmur — The patient is standing and leaning against a wall of the examining room. Use the flat diaphragm of the stethoscope exerting firm pressure. The faintest aortic diastolic murmur (listening along third left sternal border) might be detected in this seldom used position.

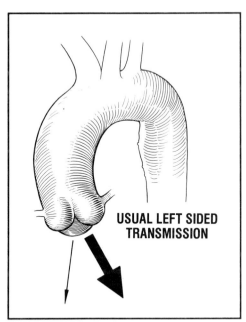

USUAL LEFT SIDED TRANSMISSION

Figure 27: Usual — The majority of murmurs of aortic regurgitation are best heard along the *left* sternal border (large arrow).

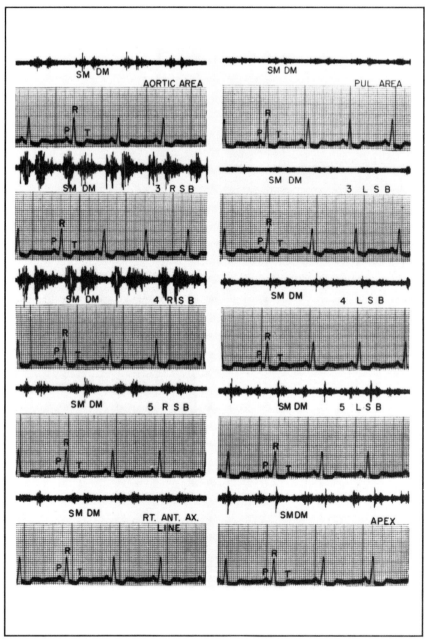

Figure 28: "Right-sided" Aortic Diastolic Murmurs — Note striking difference in intensity — louder at *right* sternal border (particularly second and third panels) compared with counterpart at left sternal border.

- This "right-sided aortic diastolic murmur" is usually associated with dilatation and rightward displacement of the aortic root (Figure 29).

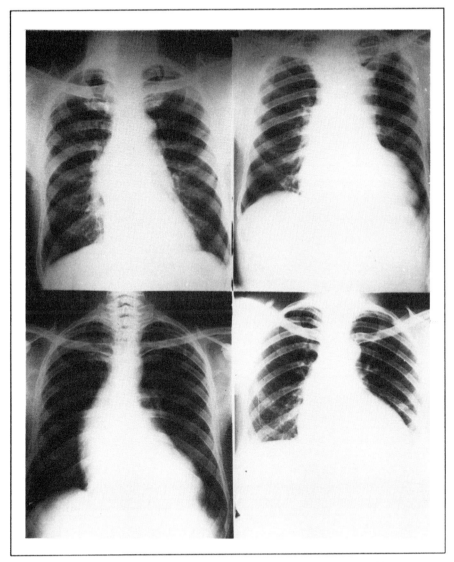

Figure 29: X-Ray Views — Four patients with right-sided aortic diastolic murmurs. Note dilatation and rightward displacement of the aortic root.

This has been associated with aortic aneurysm, aortic dissection, hypertension, arteriosclerosis, rheumatoid spondylitis, Marfan's syndrome, a variant of Marfan's, osteogenesis imperfecta, ventricular septal defect with aortic regurgitation, idiopathic, and lues (Figure 30). The key interspaces are the third and fourth right, as compared with their counterparts, the third and fourth left interspaces. The third interspaces are most likely to show the more definitive difference. An aortic diastolic murmur louder at the right sternal border than on the left immediately suggests the diagnoses just described. This valuable cardiac pearl has stood the test of time, but is frequently overlooked because we have not trained ourselves to listen to every patient along the right sternal border as well as the left. Many of the conditions that cause a right-sided murmur can also have the murmur louder on the left.

However when the "right sided aortic diastolic murmur" is present, it represents an immediate clue to one of these conditions. When the murmur is of equal intensity on both the left and right sides, one can still suspect the diagnoses as listed.

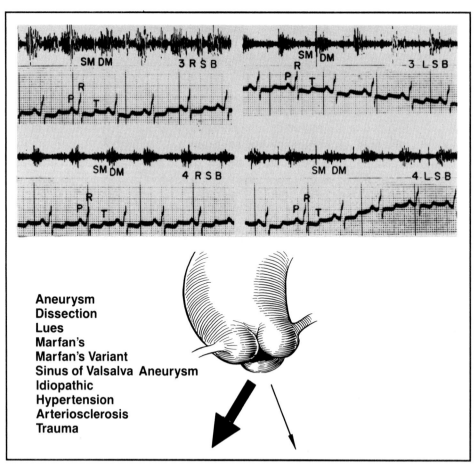

Aneurysm
Dissection
Lues
Marfan's
Marfan's Variant
Sinus of Valsalva Aneurysm
Idiopathic
Hypertension
Arteriosclerosis
Trauma

Figure 30: Some Causes of "Right-Sided" Aortic Diastolic Murmur — Note louder diastolic murmur (DM) on right sternal border (3RSB) as compared with counterpart on left (3LSB). Also note dilatation and rightward displacement of first portion of ascending aorta.

- Another cardiac pearl concerning right-sided aortic diastolic murmurs is what we term a "formula": Diastolic hypertension plus an aortic diastolic murmur plus a right-sided aortic diastolic murmur equals aneurysm and/or dissection of the first portion of the ascending aorta, as shown in the diagram.

| Diastolic Hypertension | + | Aortic Diastolic Murmur | + | "Right Sided" Aortic Diastolic Murmur | = | **Aneurysm and/or Dissection First Portion of the Ascending Aorta** |

Even when a patient has hypertension and then later develops an aortic diastolic murmur, the possibility of aneurysm and/or dissection should also be considered. The following brief anecdote is relevant:

A university professor in his sixties was admitted to the hospital with a documented diagnosis of acute myocardial infarction. He had a history of hypertension and was taking antihypertensive medication, which apparently controlled his blood pressure elevation. Approximately 10 days after the heart attack he was discharged from the hospital. Although somewhat improved, he did not return to his previous feeling of well being. Several months later he had what he described as the "flu," characterized by slight fever, generalized aching of muscles and joints, and the predominant symptom of pain in his upper back and shoulders; at times, it was so severe that it woke him at night.

He was readmitted to his hospital, and it was determined that he had some pericardial effusion, as shown on an echocardiogram, apparently thought to be of viral etiology ("flu"). He remained in the hospital a couple of weeks, during which time a repeat echocardiogram showed a decrease in the effusion.

After discharge home, convalescence was so slow that he consulted a physician friend — who in turn referred the patient to us for evaluation. On review of his problem, attention was paid to his description of the "flu." All of us have had flu, but I do not remember any patient who had pain in his upper back and shoulders to the extent described by this man. Also, he was being treated for hypertension.

On auscultation of his heart, a grade 3 aortic diastolic murmur was heard best along the third *right* sternal border; along the *left* sternal border it was a grade 1 (Figure 31). Apparently a diastolic murmur had not been detected on previous examinations. Putting several important features together, using the cardiac pearl of right-sided aortic diastolic murmur, and the "formula," the diagnosis was evident: The patient had diastolic hypertension and was under treatment for it; he had an aortic diastolic murmur; it was a "right-sided" aortic diastolic murmur. By the formula this equalled aneurysm and/or dissection of the first portion of the ascending aorta.

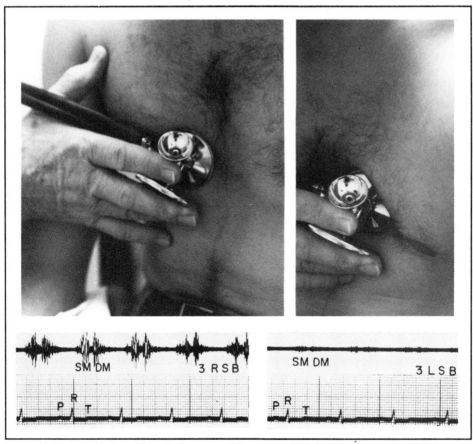

Figure 31: Right and Left — Right sided aortic diastolic murmur (DM). Note the murmur is definitely louder over the third *right* sternal border (3RSB) as compared with the third left sternal border (3LSB).

He was admitted to our hospital for surgery. He had replacement of the first portion of his ascending aorta, which was aneurysmal and dissected; his aortic valve was flail and causing significant aortic regurgitation; this was repaired, as it was decided that replacement was not necessary. The operation was life-saving to this patient.

To explain the sequence that had occurred: He indeed had an acute myocardial infarction, which was well documented on his first admission. This was caused by his aortic dissection, which involved the coronary orifices. The second admission for the "flu" was really caused by continued aortic dissection, giving him the classical back and shoulder pain (Figure 32) that can go along with aortic dissection. His pericardial effusion was blood in the pericardial sac and unrelated to the flu virus. The murmur best heard along the right sternal border had not, apparently, been detected because a stethoscope was not placed along the right sternal border, which should be routine. He thus had the components of the "formula."

It is now approximately eight years following his operation; he has returned to an asymptomatic, fruitful life, has written two books, and has made several trips to foreign countries. He represents a "reversible" type of heart disease.

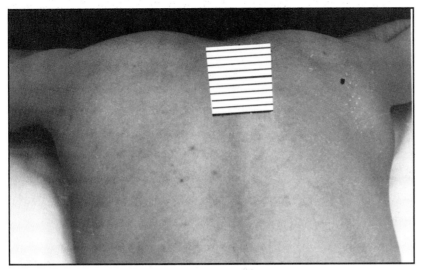

Figure 32: A Clue to Dissection — Severe pain in the upper back between the shoulder blades is a clue to aortic dissection.

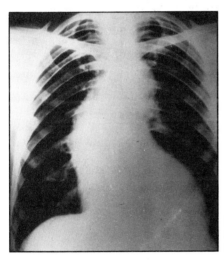

Figure 33: Dilatation and rightward displacement of the aortic root. Seeing this before listening to the patient, one can anticipate finding a right sided aortic diastolic murmur.

- **"Right-sided" murmurs of aortic regurgitation — If x-ray shows rightward displacement of the aortic root and a murmur of aortic regurgitation is present, it is most likely to be of the right-sided type.**

  Figure 33 shows a patient with rightward displacement of the aortic root. The aortic regurgitation murmur present is almost certainly to be that of a predominantly right sided type, better heard at the third and fourth *right* sternal borders than on the left.

Patients having more advanced degrees of aortic regurgitation are more likely to be aware of their arrhythmia than the person with no heart disease. They get accustomed to the "bobbing" up and down of their head. When a premature beat occurs that alters the regular prominent pulsations, they are immediately aware but tolerate it. However, if atrial fibrillation is present, producing irregular bobbing, it can be very bothersome to the patients, and they seek help to alleviate this sensation.

- **Fortunately, the majority of patients with a single aortic valvular lesion, aortic regurgitation, stenosis, or a combination of stenosis and regurgitation have a normal, *regular* sinus rhythm.**

- **If atrial fibrillation is present, suspect the possibility of a concomitant mitral valve lesion.**

Three decades ago at Georgetown University Medical Center, the first prosthetic valve (Hufnagel valve) was successfully inserted into a human (Figure 34). This artificial ball valve was placed in a patient of mine who was at the end stage of her life due to severe, advanced aortic regurgitation. Dr. Charles Hufnagel was the surgeon, and his operation had been tested in dogs for approximately six years. At that time, the heart-lung pump had not been developed, so this ball valve, made of the same material as one's toothbrush handle, was implanted in the first portion of the descending aorta. It was estimated that approximately 60% of the leak of the aortic valve (from below the prosthesis) was corrected, but of course could not alter the regurgitation coming from the upper extremities and head and neck regions. Following this successful first operation, hundreds of patients with severe aortic regurgitation were referred to our institution for surgery. Analysis of the first 100 patients with severe aortic regurgitation showed the following findings:

- They all had the typical up and down "bobbing" of the head ("yes, yes" sign) due to their aortic regurgitation.
- Many sweated frequently and even profusely, despite the fact that they were not particularly active at that time, and the air temperature was not hot. They might perspire even when it was cool or cold.
- A few had unexplained pain, tenderness to touch, over the carotid arteries (Figure 35).
- Some had unexplained mid abdominal pain.
- They all had a quick rise, "flip", or collapsing arterial pulse. The femoral arterial pulsation was even stronger than the prominent radial, brachial and carotid pulses. These complaints disappeared after surgery.

A cardiac pearl, learned from our first patient: Her femoral arterial pulse was not as strong, even though it was easily felt, as were her radial, brachial, and carotid arterial pulsations. To our surprise at surgery, she also had a mild coarctation of the aorta.

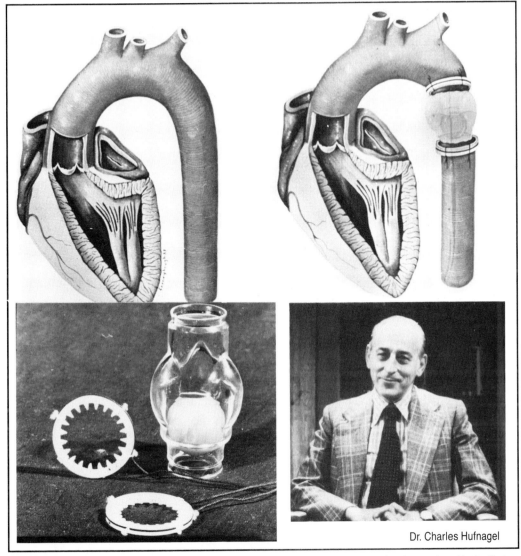

Figure 34: Hufnagel prosthetic valve for partial correction of severe aortic regurgitation. It was placed in the first portion of the descending aorta. This was the first successful prosthetic human valve for this condition.

Dr. Charles Hufnagel

- Palpate simultaneously the radial, brachial, or carotid pulse with the femoral pulse. If the carotid, brachial, or radial pulsations are better felt than the femoral, diagnose coarctation of the aorta in addition to the severe aortic regurgitation.

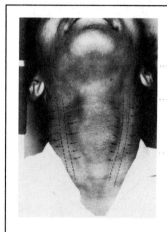

NECK PAIN — TRANSIENT

......TENDERNESS AND PAIN OVER CAROTID ARTERIES

......EXACERBATIONS AND REMISSIONS
        (UNAFFECTED BY AORTIC VALVE SURGERY)

......ETIOLOGY — UNCERTAIN

      a) PROBABLY PRODUCED IN WALL OF
         CAROTID ARTERY

      b) CAROTID PULSATIONS AGAINST TENDER
         LYMPH NODES

Figure 35: Unusual Features of Aortic Regurgitation — This patient had severe aortic regurgitation, exact cause uncertain.

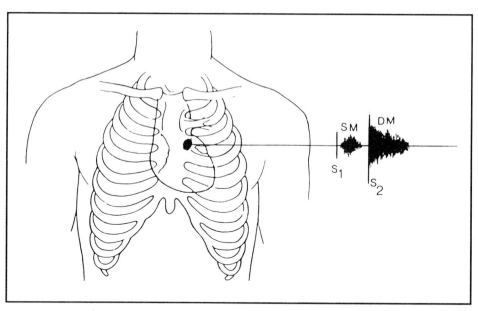

Figure 36: "To and Fro" — Systolic (SM) and diastolic (DM) murmurs of severe advanced aortic regurgitation. This patient had osteogenesis imperfecta and infective endocarditis on a porcine valve replacement.

       The easy palpation of the femoral artery is the exception to the rule for diagnosis of coarctation, since with this condition femoral pulsations are generally absent or diminished.

       On auscultation of the heart, an aortic systolic murmur followed by a typical early blowing aortic diastolic murmur was heard in each of the hundred patients — the characteristic "to and fro" murmurs of aortic regurgitation (Figures 36 and 41).

The systolic murmur was grade three or four intensity, and in some it was louder and accompanied by an aortic systolic thrill. Because of this, *aortic stenosis* was diagnosed in addition to the aortic regurgitation. However, subsequently at operation or autopsy, no stenosis was present. How to make the correct diagnosis?

- **In such a patient who has a loud aortic systolic murmur, even with a palpable systolic thrill, if on blood pressure measurement there is a wide discrepancy in the pressures, such as 160 to 170 over 40 to 30, down to zero, the patient has no stenosis — only regurgitation.**

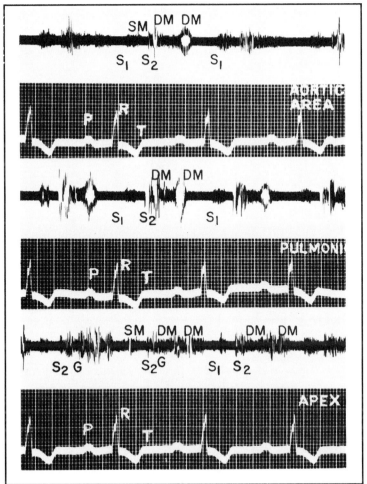

Figure 37: Austin Flint rumble (DM) at apex. Note rumble (DM) is in early as well as late diastole (presystole).

All of these first 100 patients with severe aortic regurgitation had the quick rise "flip", arterial pulse (Corrigan's, water hammer, collapsing), usually best heard along the third and fourth left sternal borders. At the lower left sternal border and apex, a different systolic murmur was heard, that of mild to moderate mitral regurgitation, most likely due to dilatation of the mitral valve ring, associated with a large, dilated and hypertrophied left ventricle. At the apex, generally in a localized spot over the left ventricle and best heard with the patient turned to the left lateral position and listening with the bell of the stethoscope over the point of maximum impulse of the left ventricle, a diastolic rumble was present. This was the Austin Flint rumbling murmur (Figures 37 and 38). Therefore, three murmurs were heard over this area.

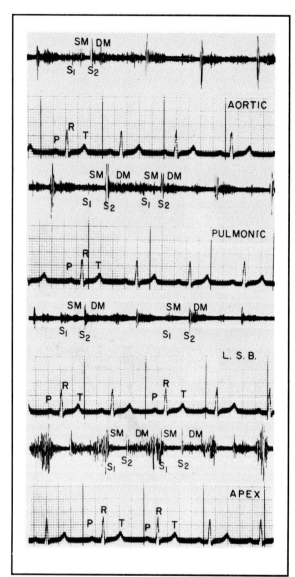

Figure 38: Austin Flint rumble (DM) at apex. Note the rumble is predominantly in presystole accentuating up to the first sound.

- **In our experience, with most severe leaks of the aortic valve, the Austin Flint rumble occurs approximately in the mid portion of systole, and often with some components in presystole. The murmurs of less advanced degrees of aortic regurgitation, though still significant, have the diastolic rumble well heard in presystole, described by Austin Flint as a "blubbering" murmur.**

It had been said that one could not tell the difference between the Austin Flint murmur and that of rheumatic mitral stenosis; however, this can be easily done.

- **When the Austin Flint murmur is heard, there is significant aortic regurgitation. Fluttering of the mitral valve is noted on the echocardiogram, and can occur not only with severe aortic regurgitation, but also with mild to moderate regurgitation.**

Patients with advanced degrees of aortic regurgitation can live longer than formerly thought. Even though left ventricular hypertrophy is present on x-ray, electrocardiogram, and echocardiogram, if these patients are asymptomatic we generally defer operation. As an example, one patient was seen 29 years ago for evaluation of his advanced aortic valve lesions, predominantly aortic regurgitation. He already had left ventricular hypertrophy, as noted on the physical examination, x-ray and electrocardiogram. When asked what his main complaint was, he said: "Nothing." Then on second thought, he said, "When I get a skip of my heart, I feel it." However, his premature ventricular contractions were not frequent, and he had adjusted to their presence. I then learned from his wife, who was present at the evaluation, that he was already on the schedule for surgery, and they had rented a room across the street from the hospital for his wife to stay while surgery and convalescence took place. In the absence of any significant symptoms, I told them that I would not have the operation; instead I recommended continued follow up care under surveillance of his private physician, plus evaluation at our hospital on a yearly basis, returning earlier if he became symptomatic.

He elected to follow this advice and went 28 years before he became symptomatic with cardiac decompensation, frequent ventricular arrhythmias, particularly multiple premature ventricular contractions, and several episodes of rapid transient atrial fibrillation (which were, of course, quite bothersome to the patient).

Finally, two years ago, he had reached the end of his rope, having extreme left ventricular dilatation and hypertrophy, and the symptoms as described. In fact, he had one episode of cardiac arrest, from which he was resuscitated. Even though it seemed to the patient's family and physicians that it was likely too late for surgery, this was done, and the patient had relief of symptoms, with an excellent salvage result.

This patient is, of course, an extreme example, but does illustrate that a patient with aortic valve disease of this type can, with appropriate medical follow-up, live longer than often thought.

The operation originally scheduled 28 years ago was to have Dr. Hufnagel's original ball valve inserted in the first portion of the descending aorta. If he had had surgery at that time, he could have died, or a few years afterwards, since repeat operation(s) would have been necessary.

It is also of interest that this patient, now over 60 years of age, has been able to perform his duties in his work as a personnel director in a hospital. At the time of the original evaluation, he had several small children, who are now adults, and in addition subsequently had another son, who is about 20 years of age. When you think about it, this child probably would not have been conceived.

- **Another Cardiac Pearl:** The quick rise or "flip" of the radial pulse may be even better detected by having the patient raise his arms over his head. This simple maneuver may make this type of pulse more evident (Figure 39).

- Prompt recognition of acute, severe aortic regurgitation, as can occur from infective endocarditis affecting the aortic valve, may be lifesaving; failure to do so is understandable, because the diastolic blood pressure may be a low normal, or be slightly or moderately reduced compared with the very low diastolic blood pressures present with severe, chronic aortic regurgitation. Also, with the acute type, the "to and fro" systolic and diastolic

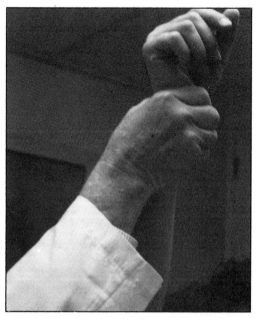

Figure 39: Aortic Regurgitation — The "quick rise" or "flip" of the radial pulse may be even better appreciated by palpation with the patient's arm elevated as shown.

murmurs heard best along the left sternal border may be shorter in duration and fainter (Figures 40 and 41). Also, the first heart sound is likely to be faint. A very important finding is a sound representing early closure of the mitral valve, occurring in the first third or mid diastole; it can even be louder than the first and/or second heart sounds, and unless the "inching" technique (as described on page 19) for timing of sounds is employed, it could be misinterpreted as either the first or second sound. This early closure of the mitral valve is due to the great leak of the aortic valve into the left ventricle, thereby closing the mitral valve prematurely — without which there would be immediate death. This precarious situation is an emergency that obviously requires early diagnosis and surgical replacement of the aortic valve.

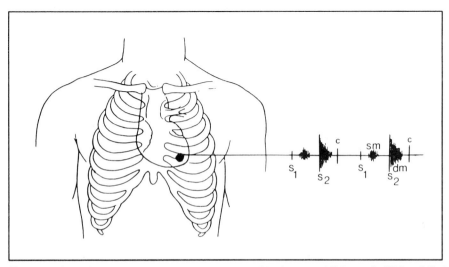

Figure 40: Acute Severe Aortic Regurgitation — Note faint first sound (S₁) systolic (SM) and diastolic (DM) murmurs and early closure sound (C) of mitral valve.

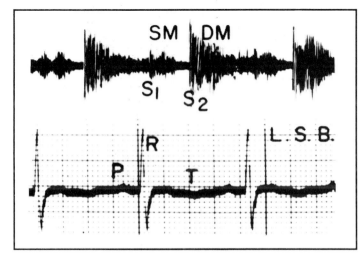

Figure 41: Advanced Regurgitation — "To and fro" murmur of advanced degrees of aortic regurgitation. These systolic (SM) and diastolic (DM) components of the murmur are best heard along the mid left sternal border. The loud diastolic murmur "tails off" immediately following the second sound (S₂).

Aortic Stenosis

The typical murmur of aortic stenosis is harsh, similar to the sound of clearing one's throat (Figures 42-51). *Aortic events are usually well heard at the apex.* Therefore the "diamond shaped" systolic murmur of aortic stenosis is usually well heard at the apex (in some, even best heard). The murmur characteristically radiates up into the supraclavicular areas of the neck, over the carotids, and suprasternal notch. I once thought that a good clinical cardiac pearl about aortic stenosis would be that the murmur would be louder over the right neck than the left. However, the cardiac pearl is that *they are heard equally well on both sides.* Also remember to listen over both clavicles; because bone is such a good transmitter of sound, it can be louder here than in the neck.

Palpation can be of great aid in the clinical diagnosis of aortic stenosis. Using both hands, the right hand is placed over the apex of the left ventricle and the left hand over the aortic area (Figure 49). A left ventricular impulse indicating hypertrophy of the left ventricle can be felt, and a palpable systolic thrill may be detected over the aortic area, the *direction* of which is toward the right neck and shoulder. A cardiac pearl relating to the palpable thrill:

- **The direction of the thrill with aortic stenosis is toward the right neck or clavicle; the direction of the thrill of pulmonic stenosis is toward the left neck and clavicle.**

The detection of a palpable thrill, which is easily identified if searched for, means that an aortic systolic murmur of at least a grade 4 intensity also will be heard; therefore the patient has aortic stenosis and can be diagnosed by palpation.

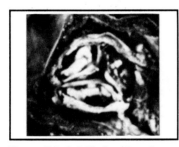

Figure 42A: Calcified aortic valve.

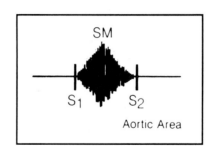

Figure 42B: Note loud, harsh, aortic systolic murmur (SM).

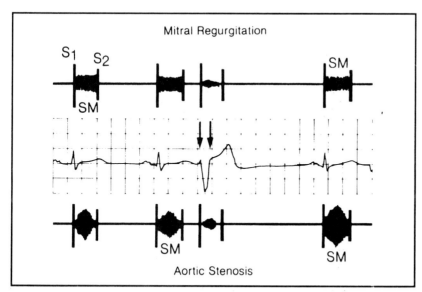

Figure 43: After Pause — Systolic murmur (SM) of mitral regurgitation remains unchanged after pause. In contrast, systolic murmur (SM) of aortic stenosis is louder after pause following premature beat.

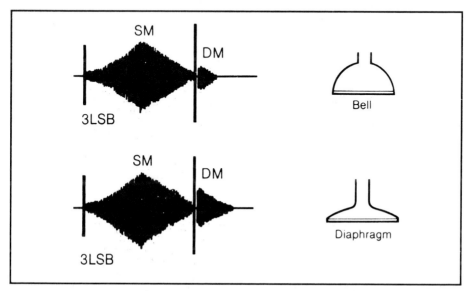

Figure 44: Faint, high-pitched, early blowing diastolic murmur of aortic regurgitation more easily heard with diaphragm of stethoscope.

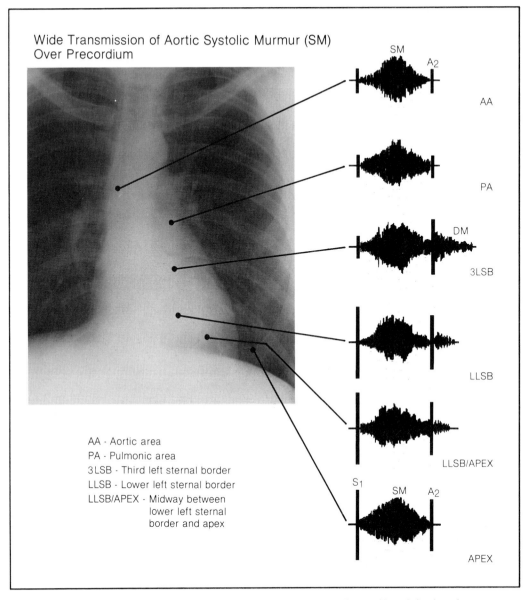

Figure 45: The aortic systolic murmur (SM) is transmitted over the precordium and heard clearly at the apex. Remember, aortic events often are heard clearly at the apex. A faint, high-pitched, early blowing diastolic murmur (DM) of aortic regurgitation also is heard best at third left sternal border (3LSB).

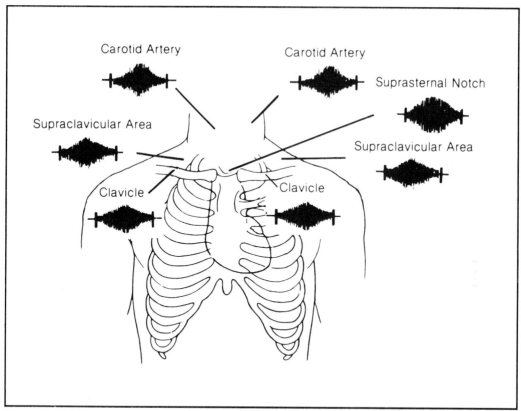

Figure 46: Wide Transmission of Systolic Murmur (SM) of Aortic Stenosis in Neck Area — Usually heard as well on left as on right. Systolic murmur is often louder over clavicles, illustrating importance of transmission by bone.

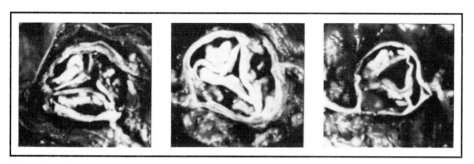

Figure 47: Three patients with calcific aortic stenosis.

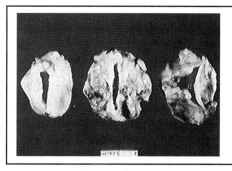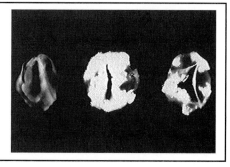

Figure 48A: Three more patients with aortic stenosis: unicuspid valve (left); bicuspid valve (middle); tricuspid aortic valve in an elderly patient with a mild degree of stenosis (right).

Figure 48B: X-ray showing calcification in each valve.

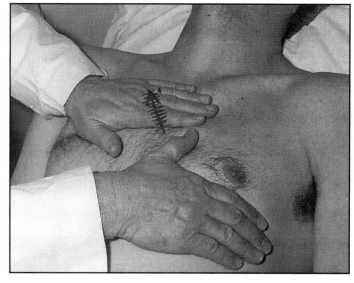

Figure 49: Two-Hand Palpation: Palpate with both hands, one on each side. Here, the right hand palpates a left ventricular impulse indicating hypertrophy. The left hand feels a systolic thrill. Two hand palpation also may provide a quick diagnosis of dextrocardia.

Also, when greeting the patient initially and paying attention to the characteristics of the radial pulse (also the brachial and carotid):

- **If it had a slow rise with a slow descent, this is consistent with aortic stenosis. If there was no quick rise or "flip" of the pulse, one could be sure no significant degree of aortic regurgitation was present.**

Therefore the diagnosis, from palpation alone, is: Significant aortic stenosis with little or no aortic regurgitation. Many times, after a complete workup in the hospital, including even cardiac catheterization, this initial clinical diagnosis from palpation is confirmed.

- **Aortic Stenosis vs Mitral Regurgitation** — To differentiate between the systolic murmur of aortic stenosis and that of mitral regurgitation, concentrate on the murmur after a pause with atrial fibrillation, or the pause after a premature beat. With aortic stenosis, the murmur increases in intensity after the pause; with mitral regurgitation, the murmur remains essentially unchanged (Figures 50 and 51).

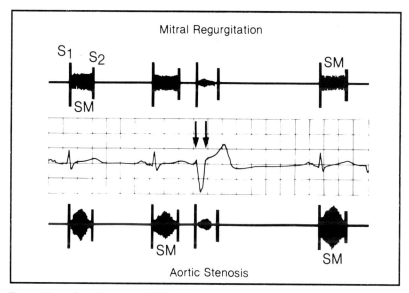

Figure 50: — Systolic murmur (SM) of mitral regurgitation remains unchanged after pause. In contrast, systolic murmur (SM) of aortic stenosis is louder after pause following premature beat.

    This pearl may even be life saving as it was for a lady in her sixties incapacitated by advanced congestive heart failure. Because of her dyspnea, she could not climb stairs and had to sleep in a chair in the upright position. Symptoms and signs of advanced heart failure persisted despite all of the usual medical therapy given. She was referred for consultation.

    When asked what she had been told concerning her heart condition she said, "I have my mitral valve damaged with mitral stenosis and regurgitation, and atrial fibrillation." On listening to her heart, atrial fibrillation was present and a grade 3 to 4 systolic murmur could be heard along the lower left sternal border and over the apex.

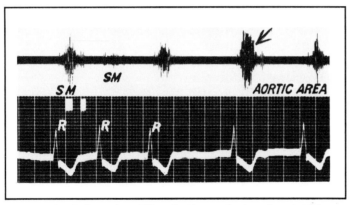

Figure 51: Aortic Stenosis — This patient has aortic stenosis and atrial fibrillation. Note beat after longer pause causes systolic murmur (SM) to get much louder (arrow).

At first it appeared that this murmur was consistent with mitral regurgitation. It was not harsh in quality. However, listening specifically after a pause of her atrial fibrillation, a definite, striking increase in her systolic murmur occurred. This was the clue that she had aortic stenosis, rather than a significant mitral valve lesion.

Cardiac catheterization was performed, which demonstrated aortic stenosis with a gradient of over 100 mm of mercury. Her stenotic valve was replaced, and she showed prompt significant improvement which has been maintained up to the present time — about nine years since her surgery.

- **Musical Murmur — If one hears a high frequency, musical, diamond shaped systolic murmur (Figure 52) heard only at the apex, immediately think of and rule out aortic stenosis.**

The patient having this type of murmur is usually elderly and has an emphysematous chest with an increase in the antero-posterior diameter. In a normal chest, this murmur is harsh in quality, like the clearing of one's throat, and is heard over the precordium rather than being localized over the lower left sternal border and/or apex. In some patients having this high frequency, musical murmur due to aortic stenosis, the typical harsh murmur can still be heard in the neck regions.

It is clinically apparent that the typical harsh, low frequency murmur of aortic stenosis can be filtered or altered by emphysematous changes and an increase in diameter to result in this musical murmur. Some have called this a "cooing dove" or "sea gull" murmur. These descriptive terms are probably best discarded, as they often cause confusion. Some physicians have used these descriptive terms to describe diastolic murmurs instead of systolic.

Having spent several decades of vacation time at my cottage on the beach, I have heard the cry of thousands of sea gulls. I can assure you that the "sea gull" murmur does not sound like the voice of a real sea gull.

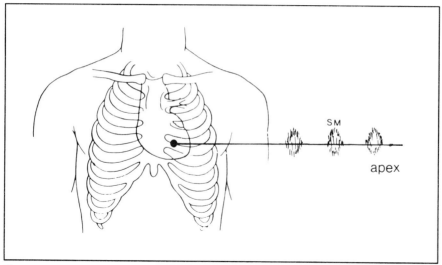

Figure 52: Musical Murmur — This is an elderly patient with emphysema and who has an increased AP diameter of the chest. A high frequency, musical systolic murmur (SM) is heard, mainly at the apex. It is important to rule out aortic stenosis in such a patient.

- **Rhythm** — **The rhythm with a *single* aortic lesion is regular (normal sinus). This applies to aortic stenosis, aortic regurgitation, or when there is both stenosis and regurgitation.**

However, if one thinks there is only a single aortic lesion (such as aortic stenosis), but atrial fibrillation is present, always look carefully for concomitant *mitral* valve involvement. A careful search may then detect, for example, an unsuspected mitral stenosis, the rumble of which may be detected only when the patient is turned to the left lateral position and the physician listens over the point of maximal impulse, with the bell of the stethoscope held lightly and barely touching the skin of the chest wall (Figure 53).

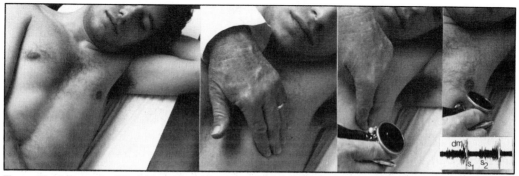

Figure 53: Listening for Mitral Stenosis — To detect a diastolic rumble (dm) of mitral stenosis, turn the patient to the left lateral position. Palpate to feel the point of maximal impulse of the left ventricle. Place the bell of the stethoscope lightly over this area (S_1 = first sound; S_2 = second sound).

- **Rheumatic Heart** — If only the aortic valve is diseased, it is most likely *not* of rheumatic etiology. A rheumatic heart generally has *two* valves involved, the aortic and the mitral.

Of course, there are some patients who have rheumatic mitral stenosis, which can be significant and symptomatic, and no aortic valve involvement is evident. However, another cardiac pearl:

- **Always look extra carefully to detect any pathology of the aortic valve, which may be only mild to moderate.**

For example, a patient (more likely a woman) who has definite mitral stenosis may at first appear to have no other valvular involvement. A lesser degree of involvement of the aortic valve might be detected only when the patient is sitting upright, leaning forward, breath held in deep expiration, and very firm pressure is exerted on the stethoscope. The flat diaphragm chest piece should be utilized rather than the bell. An early, blowing, aortic diastolic murmur may then be detected, which otherwise would be overlooked (Figure 54).

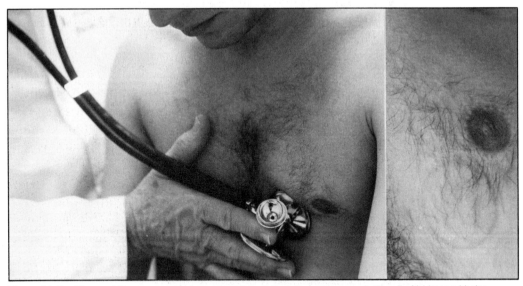

Figure 54: Position and Pressure — To detect the faintest diastolic aortic regurgitation: (Left) Listen with the patient sitting, leaning forward, with breath held in deep expiration. Exert enough pressure with the flat diaphragm of the stethoscope to leave a brief imprint of the chest piece on the skin of the chest wall (right).

- **In men, the aortic valve is most likely to be diseased. In women, it is the mitral valve.**

The reason for this difference is not clear.

50

- **Syncope — Aortic Stenosis — A patient** having symptoms of syncope, near syncope or dizziness related to severe, advanced aortic stenosis should be promptly referred for surgical valve replacement. The next episode of syncope could be the last.

- **Aortic Stenosis — Timing of Operation —** Even when a patient has documented aortic stenosis and even left ventricular hypertrophy, one can usually be more conservative in treatment if there are no symptoms related to the valve.

    Once symptoms of progressive fatigue, dyspnea, and/or dizziness occur, surgery should be considered. Surprisingly, it may take a number of years before symptoms develop.

- **Systolic Aortic Murmurs of the Elderly** — As people live longer, they often develop an aortic systolic murmur that may progressively increase in intensity, produce symptoms of fatigue, dyspnea, near syncope or syncope. This is usually caused by a tricuspid aortic valve (Figure 55).

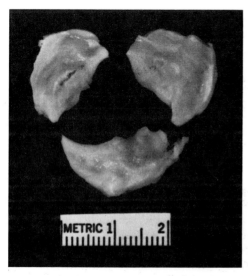

Figure 55: Severe Stenosis — This photograph shows a 3 cusp aortic valve stenosis. This is the most common type of valve stenosis in patients aged 60 to 90 years.

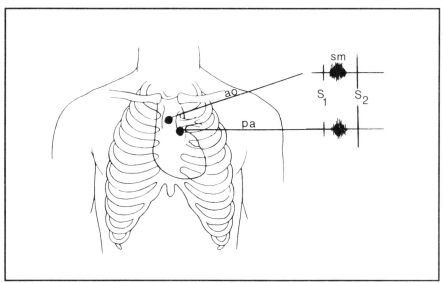

Figure 56: Innocent Systolic Murmur of the Elderly — This 84-year-old man had an "innocent systolic murmur of the elderly." He had no symptoms or signs of heart disease. He died five years later with pneumonia. Note grade 3 aortic systolic murmur which was somewhat harsh over the aortic area (ao) and had a musical quality over the pulmonic area (pa). Over a 20-year period, both before and after the development of this murmur, this patient's heart findings remained unchanged.

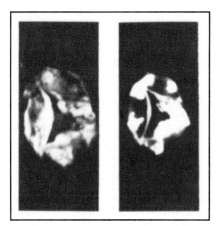

Figures 57 and 58: Tricuspid Aortic Valve — Figure on the left shows a 3 cusp aortic valve in an elderly patient with a mild degree of stenosis. Figure on the right shows an x-ray view of the same valve and reveals calcification.

Other elderly people (ages 60 to 90 +) develop an aortic systolic murmur due to a mild to moderate degree of sclerosis or stenosis. Calcium deposits of varying degree occur on the valve, but may not affect its function and the patient may have no symptoms. This murmur is termed "innocent systolic aortic murmur of the elderly" (Figure 56). Usually no treatment is required, nor is heart catheterization necessary.

The pathology of valves such as those shown in Figures 57 and 58 shows some dense sclerotic changes with calcification of portions of the three leaflet aortic valve. The commissures are not fused at their junction with the aortic ring. Although a murmur of grade 3 or less may have been heard in a patient with such a valve, no symptoms may be present. Some patients also have a faint grade 1 or 2 aortic diastolic murmur. The electrocardiogram and the heart x-ray may show no left ventricular hypertrophy. An innocent murmur of the elderly (more likely in males) may continue a benign course for years; on the other hand, progression can gradually occur and cause symptoms.

- **Sometimes, unexplained GI bleeding occurs in patients with aortic stenosis.**

    In the 1950s and 1960s, many patients with lesions of the aortic valve were evaluated for possible valve surgery at Georgetown University Hospital. As I recall, about five patients with aortic stenosis also had gastrointestinal bleeding. Workup of these patients failed to reveal any specific etiology such as ulcer, varices, gastritis or esophagitis. Following operation for aortic stenosis, the bleeding was alleviated. Similar cases have been reported from other areas of the country. Often, no explanation was found; however a few of the patients with gastrointestinal bleeding were subsequently found to have one of the GI lesions mentioned above.

- **Physical Signs of Supravalvular Aortic Stenosis — Figure 59 shows characteristic facies of a boy with supravalvular aortic stenosis.**

    It is interesting that a patient with this problem has enough look-alikes to think they might be members of the same family. Note the large mouth, large lips, prominent teeth in poor alignment, receding chin and eyes that are more widely set apart than usual. In many, the carotid artery pulsations are stronger on the right than the left. A typical harsh aortic systolic murmur is present, but the aortic ejection sound and aortic diastolic murmur are absent.

- **Congenital Aortic Stenosis — A *unicuspid aortic valve* stenosis is the most common congenital valvular lesion that causes symptoms in patients under the age of six; it is rarely found in adults.**

- **Bicuspid Aortic Valve — From ages 6 to approximately 60, bicuspid aortic valve is the most likely cause of aortic stenosis, and ranks second only to mitral valve prolapse as the most common valvular lesion.**

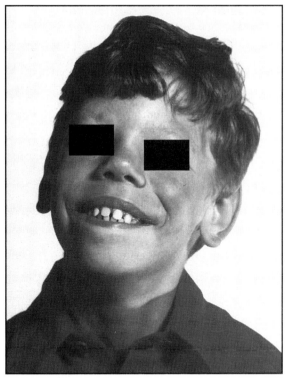

Figure 59: Signs of Supravalvular Stenosis — Characteristic facies of boy with congenital supravalvular aortic stenosis.

For example, if aortic stenosis is diagnosed in a man aged 55 and it is a single valvular lesion, the diagnosis in the great majority of patients will be congenital bicuspid aortic valve. Calcification of the valve will be present in virtually 100% of these patients.

After the age of 60, the most common cause of aortic stenosis is not congenital in origin, but rather a three leaflet (tricuspid) aortic valve.

Using the above information, the clinical diagnosis of the specific valve lesion's morphology can be accurately made. Also, remember this cardiac pearl:

- **If the aortic valve is involved as a *single* lesion, the heart rhythm is regular; if atrial fibrillation is present, always suspect and rule out concomitant mitral valve pathology.**

The patient with bicuspid aortic valve stenosis may have no symptoms. With more advanced degrees of stenosis, dizziness, near syncope or syncope, dyspnea, and fatigue can occur; a significantly loud aortic systolic murmur also would be present to alert the examining physician to this possibility. If dizziness or syncope is present and stenosis of the aortic valve is the diagnosis, it is imperative that prompt surgical replacement of the valve be performed; delay may be too late to prevent the sudden death due to ventricular fibrillation in such patients.

It is of great importance to differentiate the murmur of congenital aortic stenosis from an innocent systolic murmur (see page 102). Early diagnosis can be readily accomplished in the physician's office.

The auscultatory findings in a patient with a congenital bicuspid aortic valve represent a spectrum as shown in Figure 61. Most commonly, an early to mid-systolic murmur of grade 1 to 3 intensity is present. Frequently it has a harsh quality similar to the sound of clearing one's throat. In some, an early blowing, high frequency aortic diastolic murmur of grade 1 to 3 is heard. Firm pressure on the stethoscope's flat diaphragm chest piece should always be used to best detect this diastolic murmur, listening along the left sternal border, with the patient sitting upright, leaning forward, and breath held in deep expiration.

Since aortic events are usually well heard at the apex, the systolic murmur of aortic stenosis may be detected from the aortic area to the apex (Figure 60). This is also true of the aortic ejection sound that is another key to this condition (Figure 61).

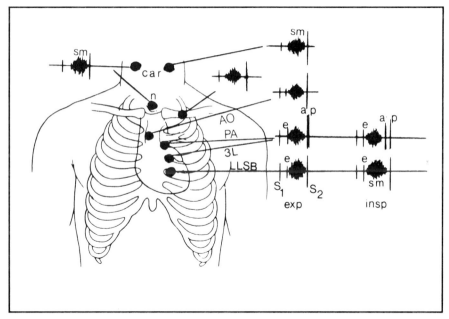

Figure 60: Aortic Stenosis — A 56-year-old man who has a congenital bicuspid aortic valve. The ejection sound (e) is unchanged by respiration and is the same over the pulmonic area (PA), third left sternal border (3L), and at the lower left sternal border (LLSB). Murmur and ejection sound are also well heard at the apex. The ejection sound is not eliminated with firm pressure of the stethoscope, as should be the case with an atrial gallop. Note the wide transmission of the systolic murmur (sm) over the precordium and neck areas (car). Normal splitting of the second sound (a-p) is heard over the pulmonic area and third left sternal border. n = suprasternal notch, CAR = carotid artery.

- **The ejection sound is a hallmark of a congenital bicuspid aortic valve and occurs with "doming" of the valve in early systole. It, too, as with the systolic murmur, is generally well heard from the apex to the aortic area (Figure 60). It does not diminish in intensity with inspiration (as can occur with the ejection sound of congenital pulmonic stenosis).**

     If severe aortic stenosis is present, one readily hears a loud (grade 4 to 6) precordial murmur. However, aortic stenosis of a mild to moderate degree can easily be overlooked on a cursory physical examination, especially if the examining physician is not listening specifically for the tell-tale findings of an ejection sound and a systolic murmur. It is also worthwhile to remember that an athlete's body build (large frame, heavy weight, and highly developed chest musculature) can diminish the intensity of sounds and murmurs heard with the stethoscope. In contrast, murmurs in children, young people, and athletes with thin chests will be more readily detected.

     With increasing severity of stenosis due to a congenital bicuspid aortic valve, the systolic murmur usually becomes louder, harsher, and longer in duration (Figure 61). It may be well heard in the neck, supraclavicular area, and over the carotids. An aortic diastolic murmur is not an unexpected finding.

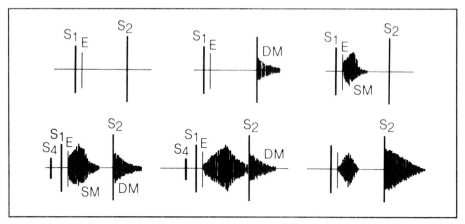

Figure 61: The spectrum of possible findings on auscultation of the congenital bicuspid aortic valve vary from only an ejection sound (E) *(no murmur)* to a systolic murmur (SM), or a diastolic murmur (DM), or combinations of both. The murmurs also are variable in intensity. An atrial sound (S_4) is likely to be present with more severe degrees of stenosis.

S_1 – First heart sound

S_2 – Second heart sound

- **It is of interest that, as part of the spectrum of findings in congenital bicuspid aortic valve, aortic regurgitation rather than stenosis may be the dominant lesion and in perhaps 5% of cases it may be of an advanced, severe degree. In some patients, no murmur is present, with only the ejection sound giving a clue to the correct diagnosis.**

Most people who have a congenital bicuspid aortic valve previously undetected would have mild to moderate degrees of stenosis. Can such a patient, asymptomatic and having a moderate degree of aortic stenosis, die suddenly? Yes; for example, I recall a 15-year-old boy who had only a moderate degree of aortic stenosis documented by cardiac catheterization. While playfully wrestling with a friend on a beach, he died suddenly. This can also occur, of course, in strenuous sports such as football, basketball, track, swimming, wrestling and others. An athlete having this type of congenital bicuspid aortic valve should be spotted during the screening evaluation; the systolic murmur and the typical ejection sound are the clues.

In contrast, an innocent murmur would have no ejection sound, and would be associated with a normal electrocardiogram and chest x-ray.

Even if the patient with a bicuspid aortic valve is asymptomatic, the electrocardiogram might show abnormalities such as left axis deviation and some increase in voltage over the left ventricle, indicating left ventricular hypertrophy. An x-ray might show some post-stenotic dilatation of the ascending aorta or other variant from normal. Such a patient would then, of course, have additional tests, including an echocardiogram and possibly cardiac catheterization to establish the diagnosis.

Chest Pain

- **If possible, try to obtain an electrocardiogram while the patient still has the chest pain
or discomfort.**

    If a patient has coronary artery disease, this may show ischemic changes that
otherwise are not present on the electrocardiogram. Therefore, when a patient first
comes in to the office or Emergency Room, if the complaint is chest pain and the
patient states that he or she is still having it, be sure to do the ECG as one of the initial
steps because the pain may be transient; if one waits until after a more detailed
history, the opportune time might be missed.

    Also helpful is to have the patient have an electrocardiogram during any
arrhythmia or palpitation or other symptoms of which he complains. This may be of
great help in identifying the problem. Also, instruct the patient that, with the onset of
any arrhythmia, he or she should promptly come to the office or Emergency Room to
have an electrocardiogram.

- **Pain of Myocardial Infarction — The
classic pain of acute myocardial infarction is
a severe precordial substernal discomfort
that radiates up to the left shoulder and then
down the left arm and along the *inside* of the
arm rather than the outside (Figure 62).**

    At times, both the right and left arms are involved with the radiation of the
pain, and in rare patients the pain is more noticeable in the right arm than the left.
The pain also may radiate up into the neck, more likely the left, but sometimes the
right or both sides of the neck. Occasionally the pain seems to be localized in the jaw,
making the patient think that this is pain in a tooth. I remember one cardiologist who
experienced pain in his tooth. He consulted his dentist who made the correct diagnosis
of acute myocardial infarction. On questioning the dentist he said that the pain from a
diseased tooth would have been in a different locale.

    In describing the classic type of chest pain from myocardial infarction, I've had
many patients describe it as a feeling like "an elephant stepped on my chest." A variant
of this was a patient who was presented to me as an unknown at a conference at the
University of Arizona. The patient described substernal precordial pain and being an
Arizona cowboy he gave the descriptive analogy of not an elephant but that of a "lasso
around my chest that was pulling tighter and tighter."

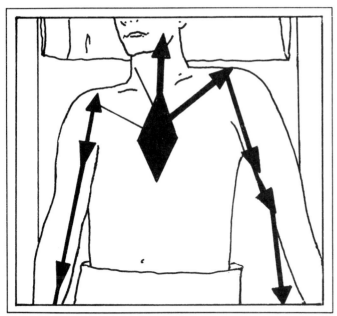

Figure 62: Radiation of coronary ischemic chest pain of acute myocardial infarction.

Sweating frequently accompanies the more severe pain of an acute myocardial infarction. Nausea and vomiting also may be present. The patient cannot seem to find a position where there is relief from the pain.

A patient with such symptoms should be admitted to an Intensive Care Unit and treated as an acute myocardial infarction, even though the initial electrocardiogram and enzymes are not diagnostic. Serial electrocardiograms and enzyme determinations are sometimes necessary to document the diagnosis.

- **Asking the Right Questions** — **To elicit a description of the typical pain caused by myocardial ischemia, ask the question, "What happens if you walk briskly up a hill, against the wind, in cold weather?"**

The patient may pause and then state, "Nothing", or "I get some shortness of breath." Does anything else happen? "Yes, I get a pressure or tightness here" (and the patient may put his hand or fist over the midportion of his sternal area). The patient may not use the word pain, but rather "pressure" or "burning," or simply "discomfort," particularly if the symptom is not severe. Some patients may only note this typical discomfort of angina pectoris after they have eaten a large meal and then walk up a hill, against the wind, in cold weather.

Be careful not to suggest to the patient that pain or discomfort might occur with this situation. That's why the question is put, "What happens if…etc." rather than saying, "Do you get pain or discomfort…etc."

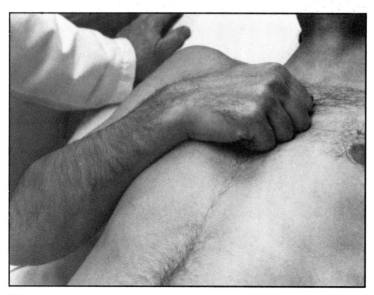

Figure 63: Levine's Sign — The patient, while describing his symptom of coronary ischemic chest pain, may make a fist with his hand and press over his substernal area. This is Levine's Sign, described by the late Samuel A. Levine of Boston (see next figure).

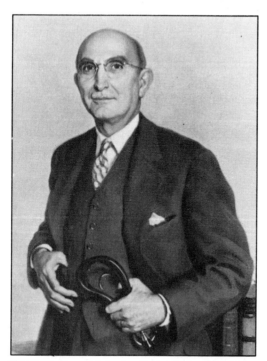

Figure 64: Samuel A. Levine, M.D., of Peter Bent Brigham Hospital, Boston. He was one of the world's leading cardiologists of his time.

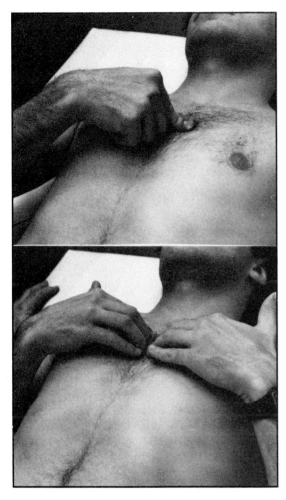

Figure 65: Variant of Levine's Sign of coronary ischemic pain. The patient may point and press with one or more fingers (top) or press with the fingers of both hands over the precordium.

- **Levine's Sign** — **A patient describing substernal chest pain or discomfort often clenches his or her fist and presses over the midsubsternal area (Figure 63). This is known as Levine's sign, named after the late Samuel A. Levine of Boston (Figure 64).**

As a variant of this sign, the patient may press over this area with the extended fingers of both hands; less commonly, the patient points and presses with one finger (usually the index finger) over the substernal area in describing the discomfort or pain (Figure 65).

An unfortunate example of this condition was my wife's brother. He had chest pain and went to the Emergency Room of his local hospital. The electrocardiogram was normal and he was allowed to go home. On arriving back home he telephoned me and related the episode of chest pain, which was typical of acute myocardial infarction, localized in the substernal area. He also said that he was pretty sure "that this was not coronary pain because it did not run down my arm." On hearing his description of the pain, I advised him to immediately go back to the hospital for admission, repeat electrocardiogram, enzymes, and for observation. He promptly got in his automobile and was driven only one block from his home when he had cardiac arrest and expired from an acute myocardial infarction. He was 39 years of age, but did have several risk factors that predisposed to coronary artery disease.

- **Pain Between the Shoulders — Chest pain more localized in the shoulders or between the shoulder blades in the back should alert one to the possibility of aortic dissection (Figure 66).**

    Although the pain of acute myocardial infarction can indeed radiate to this area in the back, the localization of the pain in the shoulder region and the back also is very consistent with the pain caused by rupture of the aorta. Be especially suspicious if the electrocardiogram does not indicate myocardial infarction.

    I remember one physician/patient who had no substernal or precordial pain, but only a pain between the shoulder blades. At first he suspected that he had an aortic dissection, but it turned out to be an acute myocardial infarction. During his convalescence, he had recurrence of mild pain, again localized to the area between the shoulders, and with no precordial component.

- **Atypical Pain of Myocardial Infarction — Coronary pain can occur in atypical locations: Between the shoulder blades, in the thumbs, in the right upper quadrant.**

    I recall one patient, a surgeon who had performed more gallbladder operations than probably any other surgeon in his community. One day he complained of pain in his right upper quadrant (Figure 67). He was under the impression that the pain was being caused by his gallbladder and arranged for a gallbladder test the following morning. At a chance meeting in the hall of the hospital, he related this story to me and I suggested a cardiology examination. On such examination there was no evidence of any acute manifestation of coronary disease. Electrocardiogram and enzyme studies were normal. However, he was advised to cancel the gallbladder test and to have a repeat electrocardiogram and enzyme studies the next morning. The following morning he again had a recurrence of moderate distress over his right upper quadrant. Repeat electrocardiogram showed an acute myocardial infarction. At no time did he have typical pain above the diaphragm. His course was uncomplicated in the hospital, except for one brief episode of discomfort — again the pain was in the right upper quadrant, the gallbladder region. A gallbladder series was obtained at a later date and it was normal.

    Another example of pain due to myocardial infarction involved the father-in-law of a physician colleague. His pain was localized to the thumb of each hand.

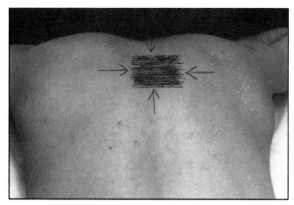

Figure 66: Dissection — Pain localized in the upper back and interscapular area can occur with aortic dissection.

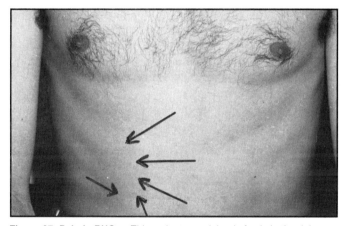

Figure 67: Pain in RUQ — This patient complained of pain in the right upper quadrant. It turned out to be an acute myocardial infarction. Gallbladder pain was initially suspected by the patient, who was a surgeon. He had no precordial pain.

Occasionally, a patient will describe the radiation of the ischemic pain from coronary artery disease as being "like an advancing tidal wave," from the substernal area to the left shoulder and then down the left arm to the fingertips. When the pain begins to subside, the "tidal wave" reverses direction back to the heart.

- **Non-Coronary Chest Pains — It is worthwhile to explain to patients the type of chest pain that generally is _not_ related to heart disease:**

- **A constant "aching" pain that might be in the substernal area and lasts all day is usually**

not caused by heart disease. Nor is pain that is present only in one position and not in others.

- **Coronary pain is not accentuated by external pressure over the precordium.**

- **Pain over the apical region of the heart or over the right anterior chest region is not typical of coronary artery pain.**

- **The fleeting, momentary pain in the chest described as a needle jab or stick, lasting only a second or two, is not heart pain.**

The patient can be reassured that these types of pain are not significant and not signs of a new or recurrent coronary artery disease.

It is reassuring to tell patients who have had an acute myocardial infarction and are returning home — back to physical activities and their occupation — about these noncoronary chest pains. Point out that it will be natural for them to look for pain, and almost certainly some of the pains described will occur. If patients are aware of them and are reassured, unnecessary fears and anxieties can be prevented.

- **Pain in the left arm can be misinterpreted as being of coronary origin. One such pain is similar to that caused when a blood pressure cuff is left inflated too long and the radial pulse is occluded.**

One can occlude his own radial pulse by moving the arm backwards and rotating it in such a manner that there is interference of the arterial blood supply to the left arm. Occasionally a patient will sleep in such a position that his or her left arm is extended and partially occluding the arterial pulse. The pain from this condition can simulate the arm pain from coronary ischemic pain. One such patient is recalled who would have pain lasting for hours or days; it extended from the shoulders down his left arm to the hand. To further complicate the picture, the patient also had a hiatal hernia. At first, coronary artery disease was suspected, but an extensive cardiovascular workup was negative. A detailed history revealed that the patient often awoke with the pain, which led to questions about the positioning of his arms while sleeping. His answers indicated that he might be occluding the arterial blood supply to his arm in his sleep. The patient was advised to sleep in a position where his arms and shoulder were not in a position to occlude the pulse. This solved his problem.

- **Pain and paresthesias involving the hands can occur during the weeks and months of convalescence after a myocardial infarction. Increased coldness and perspiration of both hands also can occur.**

These sensations and signs generally disappear with the passage of time and usually are no cause for concern to the patient.

- **Raynaud's Disease — A patient with Raynaud's Disease can have arm pain misinterpreted as coronary ischemic pain.**

If a patient complains of arm pain while driving an automobile in the winter before the heater has warmed up the car, suspect Raynaud's Disease. Such pain can be an early symptom and at first can be erroneously diagnosed as ischemic heart disease.

- **Patients with severe aortic regurgitation may have chest pain localized in the substernal area that can be so severe as to simulate acute myocardial infarction.**

I remember a West Virginia mountaineer who had severe, advanced aortic regurgitation. His bedroom was heated by a wood stove and on awakening in the morning, as he was starting the fire in the wood stove to heat up the cold bedroom, he would have onset of severe substernal precordial pain. He claimed he would set fire to an entire set of book matches and inhale the heat. This would relieve his chest pain. No electrocardiographic evidence of myocardial infarction could be found.

Miscellaneous

- **Thyrotoxicosis (Hyperthyroidism) —
There is no specific precordial murmur of
thyrotoxicosis.**

    In the past, a "scratchy" pulmonic murmur, the so-called Means-Lerman murmur (sometimes called a "crunch sound"), was identified with this condition. True, a "scratchy" early to mid-systolic murmur can be present, but the same type of murmur is heard in other conditions and is not specific for hyperthyroidism. It is probably related to increased blood flow through a hemodynamically dilated pulmonary artery.

- **Large Breasts — Listen under the breasts,
not over them.**

    When examining a woman who has large breasts (Figure 68), she can aid in the examination of the chest and in particular the left apical area by holding her

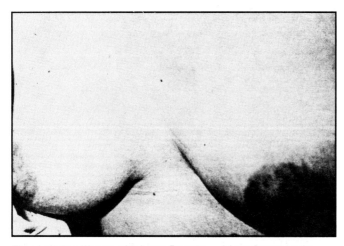

Figure 68: In a Woman with Large Breasts — A large breast can be lifted upward and away from the apical area by the physician's left hand to enable adequate auscultation. At times the patient can be requested to help in this way. Correct placement of the electrodes of the electrocardiogram can also be aided by the maneuver, if necessary.

breast upward, away from the area to be examined. This is helpful in locating the point of maximal impulse of the left ventricle, thrills, impulses of left ventricle hypertrophy, ventricular aneurysm, presystolic movement correlating with the atrial (S_4) gallop, etc. The physician can accomplish this by moving and holding the breast away from the apical area with his left hand and listening with his stethoscope in his right hand.

When an electrocardiogram is taken on a patient with large breasts, the left breast should be moved to allow accurate placement of the left precordial leads — a simple but important point, often overlooked.

• Gynecomastia and Digitalis — Occasionally a man taking digitalis may develop enlarged, tender breasts.

This is not a serious side effect; discontinuing the drug will accomplish regression, but usually this is not necessary. I have also seen some women who complained of breast tenderness after starting to take digitalis.

An innocent systolic murmur can be produced or accentuated by fever (Figure 69). It also can be the result of exercise (Figure 70).

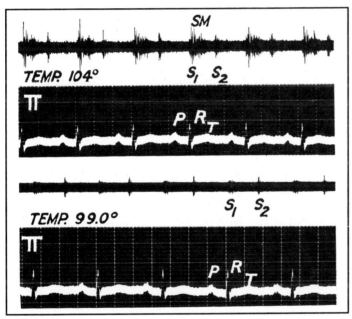

Figure 69: Fever — An innocent murmur (SM) can be produced with fever. Note absence of murmur when the patient's fever has subsided.

• "Splash" Sounds — So-called "splash" sounds can occur in patients who have a large, dilated left ventricle, such as occurs with advanced aortic regurgitation. These

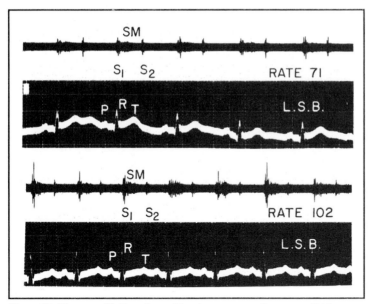

Figure 70: Murmur with Exercise — Note innocent systolic murmur (SM) becomes louder with exercise and increase in heart rate.

sounds can best be heard over the lower left sternal border and mitral area.

These high frequency sounds occurring with systole are not common and can be confusing to the physician who has not heard them before. Splash sounds in themselves do not have any serious significance.

- **Diaphragmatic Flutter — Diaphragmatic flutter is a very rare condition, usually of unknown cause, in which the diaphragm contracts rapidly, regularly and involuntarily. It is similar to a tic in other parts of the body.**

It can occur in paroxysmal form and surprisingly may produce few if any symptoms. Figure 71 is an example. However, diaphragmatic flutter sounds sometimes may be heard only when the patient is in a terminal state.

The diagnosis can be made on fluoroscopic examination and also should be easily detected on echocardiography. On fluoroscopy, the rapid, small but definite contractions are superimposed on the normal inspiratory and expiratory excursions of the diaphragm. The diaphragmatic flutter can produce sounds that can be heard over all of the chest. They are usually of low frequency and better appreciated using light pressure with the bell of the stethoscope.

The first patient with diaphragmatic flutter personally observed caused me to wonder if I were listening to two different hearts within the chest. Also the sounds can

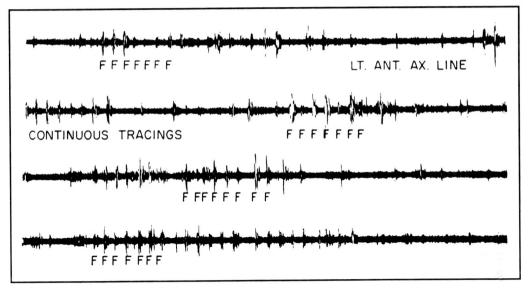

Figure 71: Diaphragmatic Flutter — Note very rapid, intermittently louder sounds (F) made by fluttering of the diaphragm, easily heard with the stethoscope.

be misinterpreted as being those of atrial flutter in addition to the normal heart sounds. I have also heard and recorded these diaphragmatic flutter sounds (Figure 72) while the patient was sleeping, which ruled out any voluntary relation by the patient.

- **Acute Mediastinal Emphysema (Hamman's Disease) — Acute mediastinal emphysema is a condition in which air from an area of lung ruptures into the anterior mediastinum. When it occurs suddenly it may be confused with an acute myocardial infarction or acute pericarditis.**

    It can be a complication of underwater swimmers — "frog men" and scuba divers. In addition to occurring spontaneously, mediastinal emphysema frequently occurs after open heart surgery and operations involving the pleura or mediastinum; it is usually self limited and transient, lasting only a few hours.

- **Auscultation can afford an immediate diagnosis of acute spontaneous mediastinal emphysema. One may hear bizarre crunching, often loud sounds over the precordium, mainly during systole and to a lesser extent in diastole (Figures 73 and 74). These sounds have been likened to a person walking on "crunchy snow." They are best heard around**

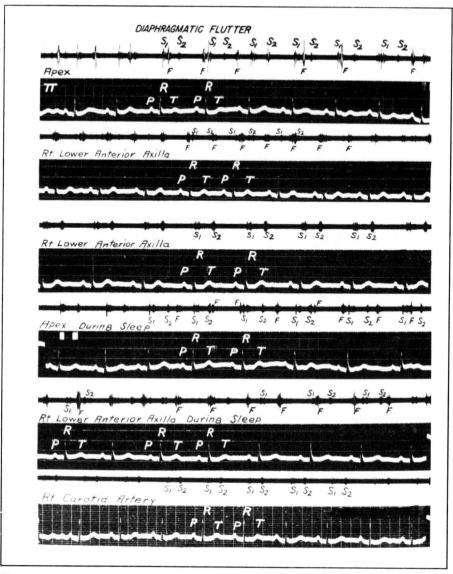

Figure 72: More Examples of Flutter — Sounds (F) easily heard with the stethoscope, produced by a fluttering of the diaphragm. Note flutter sounds also heard while patient slept (4th and 5th panels).

the lower left sternal border and apex but at times can be heard only when the person turns and lies in the left lateral position.

Occasionally the sounds are so loud that they can be heard without a stethoscope and at a distance of several feet. The patient also may be aware of these sounds and learns that a certain position or phase of respiration can bring them out, more

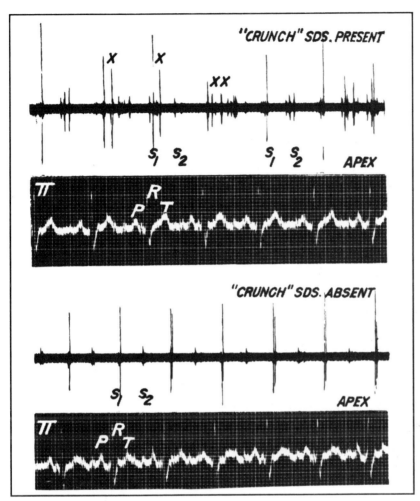

Figure 73: Acute Mediastinal Emphysema — (Upper tracing) Note bizarre sounds (X) in addition to normal sounds (S₁, S₂). Later, there are normal sounds only (lower tracing).

likely when the breath is held in inspiration or when performing a Valsalva maneuver.

The finding of air in the pleural cavity or the anterior mediastinum on x-ray can aid in the diagnosis. The electrocardiogram can be normal, but occasionally ST and T-wave changes may be present, thereby causing an erroneous diagnosis of heart disease such as pericarditis or myocardial infarction.

- **Micturition Syncope** — **Micturition syncope can occur when a man is urinating.**

A man may awaken from sleep and, still sleepy, goes to the bathroom to urinate. Postural hypotension develops, contributing to it might be some vagal stimulation coincident with straining with urination, and syncope results. The occurrence of this in women would be unusual, since they are sitting while urinating.

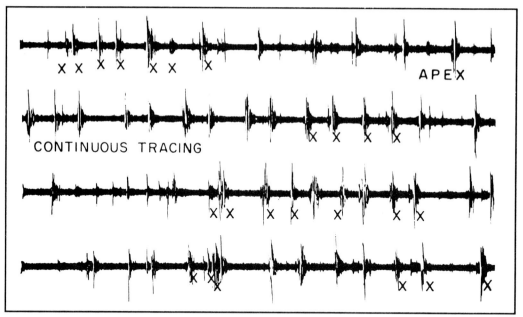

Figure 74: Another Patient with Acute Mediastinal Emphysema — Note crunch sounds (X).

- **Hyperventilation can sometimes cause symptoms similar to those of heart disease, including chest discomfort, dyspnea, dizziness, near syncope, or tachycardia.**

Illustrating this point are two patients; the first was a middle aged man who had congenital ventricular septal defect. He had a moderate sized defect, and had been asymptomatic. However, he was admitted to the Emergency Room of a local hospital when he developed chest discomfort, shortness of breath, paresthesias of both arms and hands, dizziness, and near syncope while eating in a restaurant. On examination there was no change from previous examinations. Also there was no reason why an uncomplicated ventricular septal defect should produce his symptoms.

He was instructed to hyperventilate and, sure enough, started to have symptoms similar to those he had in the restaurant. He perspired, complained of substernal chest pain, appeared anxious and had dizziness and obvious respiratory distress. Carpal spasm appeared bilaterally. Subsequently a movie was made of him again showing the same symptoms and signs due to hyperventilation. To stop the hyperventilation syndrome, he was told to look at his watch and stop breathing for every 15 seconds before he took another breath. At first this was difficult, but he did so.

Then, on repeating the purposeful breath holding alternating with breathing, one could see the reversal of all of the symptoms and signs of his hyperventilation. Subsequently this film was used to show this patient and other patients how to manage, as well as prevent, these episodes. Fortunately, the patient learned to control as well as prevent subsequent attacks.

Another patient, a 32-year-old unmarried woman, was evaluated because of what had been called "symptoms related to her mitral valve prolapse." The patient had a history of what reportedly had been documented by echocardiography to be mitral valve prolapse. Her father, who accompanied her, stated that she had recently seen her physician who again described her heart as "still clicking away." However, a careful evaluation did not reveal a systolic click or any other auscultatory evidence of mitral valve prolapse. She then had an echocardiogram at our institution, searching carefully for any evidence of mitral valve prolapse, and none was found. A follow-up examination with a repeat echocardiography was performed; again no evidence of mitral valve prolapse. During her physical examination while sitting upright on the examining table, she was asked to hyperventilate (which had been demonstrated to her). Shortly thereafter she had chest discomfort, perspiration, paresthesias of the upper extremities, and subsequent carpal spasm. Her father was present at the time of the examination; both said these were the identical symptoms that the patient had been having and had been attributing to her "mitral valve prolapse." She had been misdiagnosed as having mitral valve prolapse.

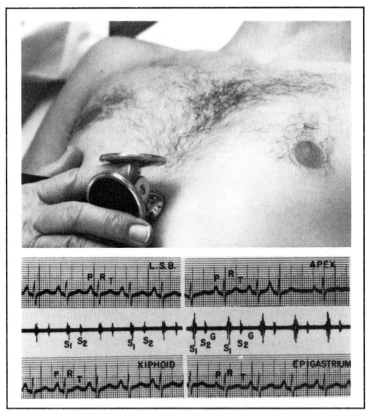

Figure 75: Xiphoid — The stethoscope is over the xiphoid (or epigastric area). A patient having an emphysematous chest might have faint sounds (S_1, S_2) heard over the precordial area (left sternal border (LSB) and apex, but well heard over the xiphoid and epigastrium. Note that a ventricular gallop (G) is heard only over the epigastric area (right lower panel).

- **An emphysematous chest with an increase in anterior-posterior (A-P) diameter can diminish the intensity of heart sounds and murmurs.**

For example, an atrial (S_4) or ventricular (S_3) gallop might not be heard over the lower left sternal border and apex. Be sure, then, to listen also over the xiphoid and epigastric areas where these sounds might be more readily heard (Figure 75).

- **The question is often asked, "How do you tell the difference between a split second sound, the opening snap of mitral stenosis, the pericardial knock sound of constrictive pericarditis, a tumor sound of atrial myxoma, a normal third heart sound, a ventricular diastolic gallop, an atrial diastolic gallop and a systolic click?" The answer is: They all sound different.**

We have high fidelity tape recordings of all of these sounds which one can listen to (individually or in a teaching conference) and one can readily learn and appreciate the difference of these sounds. Helpful also is to see a sketch of these extra sounds as shown in Figures 76 and 77.

Calcification of the mitral valve annulus, as noted on chest x-ray and fluoroscopy, was first described by the late Merrill Sosman of Boston, a master radiologist; he described the finding on fluoroscopy of the heart of a calcification resembling a letter "C" or "J". This calcified annulus can occur in some patients with mitral valve prolapse and may be related to some of the auscultatory findings of prolapse, including a systolic murmur. In other patients having the calcification no murmur is present (Figure 78).

- **Cardiac Pearl — A patient with calcification of the mitral valve annulus is more likely to have atrial fibrillation than a patient without calcification. This also applies to patients with mitral valve prolapse — those with calcification of the mitral annulus are more prone to have atrial fibrillation.**

Therefore, as might logically be expected, emboli are more likely. Anticoagulant therapy as prophylaxis should be considered in this group.

In several patients having a calcified mitral annulus, I have observed that the first heart sound is accentuated, although the P-R interval on the electrocardiogram is not short. However, a larger number of patients need to be studied before we can verify this as a "cardiac pearl." Look for it and let me know.

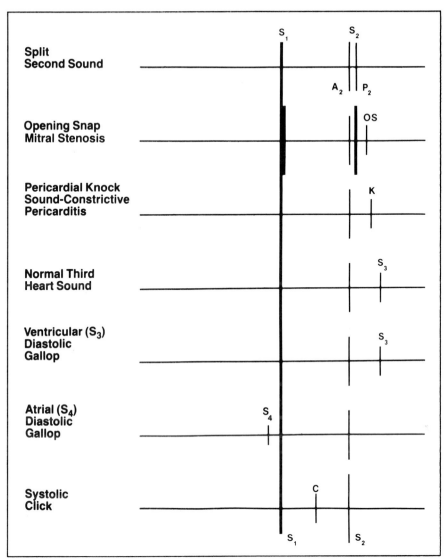

Figure 76: Differentiating Sounds — Comparison of the timing of extra sounds and events. Note that the S_1 and P_2 are accentuated with mitral stenosis. With constrictive pericarditis a pericardial knock (K) occurs later than opening snap (OS) and S_1 is not accentuated.

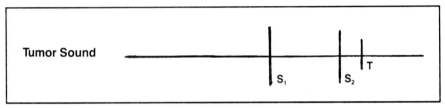

Figure 77: Myxoma — A 45-year-old man with myxoma of the left atrium. Note tumor sound (T) occurring later in timing after S_2 than the opening snap of mitral stenosis, but earlier than the normal third heart sound or S_3 gallop. The tumor sound is about the timing of a pericardial knock sound.

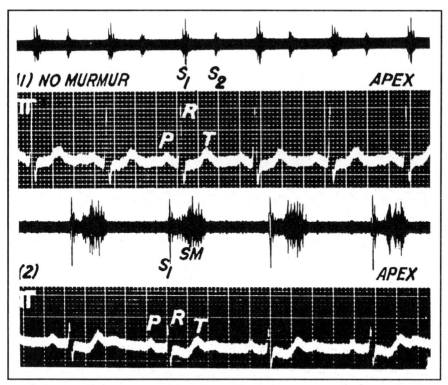

Figure 78: Calcified Annulus — Two patients with calcified mitral annulus. Patient number 1 (top panel) has no murmur. Patient number 2 (lower panel) has a late apical systolic murmur (SM) of mitral valve prolapse. The first sound (S_1) is loud even though the PR interval is not short.

- **Murmur of Stenosed Artery?** — **Can a murmur be produced by a stenosed coronary artery and be heard with the stethoscope over the precordium? Several such case reports have been reported in the literature over the past few years. However, I am skeptical of these reports. Certainly if it does occur it is extremely rare.**

    I have searched for such murmurs for a number of years and have yet to find one that is continuous or diastolic.

- **When examining a patient and asking that he or she change from the supine position to that of sitting, remember that the patient may be very uncomfortable with the legs still extended straight on the bed or examining table. Simply ask the patient to sit with legs bent and dangling over the side, which is comfortable (Figure 79).**

76

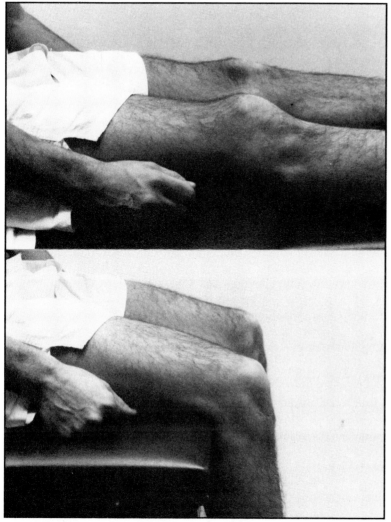

Figure 79: Comfort — When examining a patient in the sitting position, it is uncomfortable for him or her to sit with legs extended on the examining table (top); instead, it is natural and comfortable to sit with the knees bent and legs dangling over the side (bottom).

- **Ear Lobes** — **At times you may see movement of the patient's ear lobes coincident with systole. This should immediately suggest two possible causes: severe aortic regurgitation or severe tricuspid regurgitation.**

In each instance, the movement of the ears reflects the transmitted impulse from the carotid artery (aortic regurgitation) or the jugular vein (tricuspid regurgitation).

- **Carcinoid Tumor** — **When flushing occurs or the patient has persistent violaceous or erythematous facial flushing, then the carcinoid tumor of the intestine has metastasized to the liver.**

A patient was evaluated because of the finding of a systolic murmur over the pulmonic area. He described flushing of his face when he ate his breakfast and his noonday meal, but not with his evening meal. The next morning, however, he would again flush with eating. We watched as the patient ate his usual breakfast; indeed, his face flushed. To explain the lack of flushing at the evening meal, it was postulated that his serotonin stores in the body had been depleted by the evening, but were replenished during the night.

The carcinoid syndrome can also cause a reddish-pink facial hue, as if a person were blushing. I recall examining a woman who had such a coloration constantly. Evaluation was requested because of the presence of a systolic murmur. The murmur was diagnosed as a mild degree of obstruction of the pulmonic valve. She was asked whether she had been out in the sun, because her facial appearance simulated a sunburn. She said no, she had not been out in the sun at all. She had a variant of the violaceous facial hue that can occur with a carcinoid.

The serotonin in the bloodstream of patients with the carcinoid syndrome can cause scarring of the pulmonic valve, producing the pulmonic systolic murmur.

- **Bizarre Musical Murmurs** — **The presence of a transvenous pacemaker across a tricuspid valve can occasionally produce peculiar, bizarre musical murmurs.**

I recall hearing such a murmur in a patient who had just had a pacemaker inserted. The sounds, heard in both systole and diastole, sounded like the "croaking of a frog". On repositioning of the catheter, the sounds disappeared.

In other patients, the catheter across any valve may cause a sound that simulates the systolic "whoop" of mitral valve prolapse. Again, it is related to the catheter position, and the sound disappears on removal or repositioning of the catheter.

- **Thromboembolism** — **Thrombophlebitis is most likely to occur in the calf (more common) or pelvic veins. Congestive heart failure predisposes. Prolonged pressure over the calf muscles also predisposes.**

Several factors are important. (A) Avoid stockings that have the top portion of the elastic constricting at the calf level. Make sure that the elastic is above the calf, or wear ankle length socks (Figure 80). (B) Personally observed have been patients, even without heart disease, who have developed thrombophlebitis from their occupational

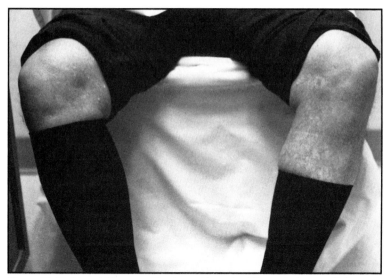

Figure 80: Right and Wrong — Elastic stockings should have their top well above the calf (left, correct way). Right, wrong way: The top of the stocking compresses the mid calf of the patient. This can predispose to phlebitis, especially in the patient having heart disease with cardiac decompensation.

duties: An air conditioning installer who had to work in cramped positions with his knees and hips bent; another, a first class pilot with a major airline who, on a long distance overseas flight, developed acute disability with chest pain and shortness of breath. The co-pilot had to take over. The pilot had acute thrombophlebitis of a calf vein with pulmonary emboli. It was determined that his phlebitis resulted from his calf resting on a new seat in the cockpit of the plane; prolonged pressure over the calf impeded venous flow, resulting in clotting and thrombosis.

Further emphasizing the need to move and exercise the leg muscles when travelling was a physician acquaintance and patient, who drove nonstop from upstate New York to Washington, D.C. and developed thrombophlebitis in the right calf region; a pulmonary embolus occurred requiring emergency hospital admission. He had kept his leg in the same position on the accelerator pedal. He did not have heart disease. Cardiac pearl: "An ounce of prevention." Break up prolonged automobile trips by stopping at intervals, such as every hour, getting out of the car and walking around.

On an airplane, get an aisle seat if possible and get up and walk at intervals. During travel, remember to occasionally wiggle your feet and move your legs at intervals.

• Varicose Veins — Causes, particularly in women, are childbearing and inheritance.

Test for Thrombophlebitis — Palpation over each calf of the lower extremities should be a routine on every physical examination. A simple but rewarding cardiac pearl in this aspect of the physical examination is to divert the patient's attention away from the fact that your fingers are palpating the calf region, by simply asking a question such as, "Do you get short of breath?" or "What do you eat for breakfast?" **While the patient is talking and answering the question, the physician's fingers are palpating the calf of both extremities. If the patient stops in the middle of answering a question and says, "Oh, that hurts", this is consistent with the diagnosis of thrombophlebitis.**

On the other hand, if the patient's attention is not diverted but is focused on the palpation of the calves and you say, "Does this hurt?", the patient often may say, "Well, yes that hurts", or "yes, a little bit."

Such an answer is more difficult to evaluate than the definite discomfort or pain that occurred when the attention was diverted.

- **Boot Phlebitis** — **As part of today's fashion, a number of women wear boots (Figure 81). Unfortunately some of these have a length that encompasses the calves of the legs. Sometimes the boots are so tight that thrombophlebitis can result. This is more likely to occur in women who are obese and have large legs and in women who may not be obese but have large calf muscles. Women who wear boots should be cautioned about this complication.**

It is of interest that several decades ago there was controversy as to whether anticoagulants were indicated for patients having atrial fibrillation.

However, recent analysis showed that patients who have atrial fibrillation will be less prone to thromboembolic events if they are on warfarin (Coumadin) or aspirin. Of course, contraindications to anticoagulant administration should be checked before use of these drugs.

- **Stroke** — **The incidence of stroke associated with atrial fibrillation can be reduced by the use of anticoagulants such as warfarin (Coumadin) and aspirin. When warfarin is contraindicated, aspirin appears to be a good substitute.**

With life expectancy increasing, more patients will have atrial fibrillation; the above pearl will be even more apropos.

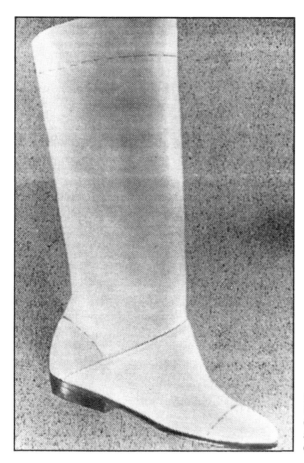

Figure 81: Tight Boots — Patients with very large calf muscles (or enlargement due to obesity) should avoid wearing boots that constrict and compress the calves — thrombophlebitis can result.

Stroke represents one of the most serious and devastating complications that can occur in cardiovascular disease. Recovery and improvement, if this occurs, is generally slow compared with other diseases. However, if we see some improvement, even though slight, it is a sign that additional improvement is possible, but again not likely to be rapid. Since patients who have suffered a stroke are so depressed and discouraged, they need to know and should be told that improvement can take place, but *slowly;* if it occurs more quickly, good. It is a bonus.

Infective Endocarditis

Following simple dental procedures such as cleaning, filling, and extractions, infective endocarditis can occur and involve a heart valve. For example, an asymptomatic patient having a congenital bicuspid aortic valve can, as a result of infective endocarditis, promptly produce a wide open, severe aortic regurgitation requiring valve replacement.

- **Cardiac Pearl — Such a patient would almost certainly have an aortic ejection sound heard at the apex as well as at the base, in addition possibly a faint aortic diastolic murmur which would be heard most likely if the patient is sitting upright, leaning forward, breath held in deep expiration, and if enough pressure is exerted on the diaphragm of the stethoscope against the chest wall to produce an imprint on the skin.**

  If such a patient's faint murmur is diagnosed and appropriate prophylaxis (as suggested by the American Heart Association) given, this unfortunate sequence of events might be prevented.

- **Antibiotic prophylaxis as outlined by the American Heart Association is indicated not only for extractions of teeth but also for the simple procedures of cleaning and/or filling. Infective endocarditis has been definitely documented to occur with these simpler procedures.**

- **Antibiotic prophylaxis should also be given to patients with valvular heart disease. Infective endocarditis can also affect valves replaced at surgery.**

- **Mitral Valve Prolapse — It has been my policy to give antibiotic prophylaxis to *all* patients with mitral valve prolapse — those**

having a click or clicks, as well as those patients with a systolic murmur.

Some authorities recommend prophylaxis only for patients with mitral valve prolapse who have a systolic murmur. They feel it is not necessary for those who have a click or clicks, but no murmur. I disagree with this because I can cite many patients with mitral valve prolapse who have transient murmurs as well as clicks. Personally observed have been patients who have had proven infective endocarditis who had only a single click or clicks and never had a systolic murmur detected on careful auscultation. It is also well known that a patient on one occasion may have only a click or clicks, whereas at other times a typical late apical systolic murmur is present, and readily heard. Occasionally, no murmur or clicks are detected.

Fortunately and reassuring, over the past several decades I have not seen significant complications in patients who received antibiotic prophylaxis.

Antibiotic Prophylaxis Against Bacterial Endocarditis

For Dental/Oral/Upper Respiratory Tract Procedures

I. Standard Regimen In Patients At Risk (includes those with prosthetic heart valves and other high risk patients):

Amoxicillin 3.0 g orally one hour before procedure, then 1.5 g six hours after initial dose.*

For amoxicillin/penicillin-allergic patients:

Erythromycin ethylsuccinate 800 mg or erythromycin stearate 1.0 g orally 2 hours before a procedure, then one-half the dose 6 hours after the initial administration.*

—OR—

Clindamycin 300 mg orally 1 hour before a procedure and 150 mg 6 hours after initial dose.*

II. Alternate Prophylactic Regimens For Dental/Oral/Upper Respiratory Tract Procedures In Patients At Risk:

A. For patients unable to take oral medications:

Ampicillin 2.0 g IV (or IM) 30 minutes before procedure, then ampicillin 1.0 g IV (or IM) OR amoxicillin 1.5 g orally 6 hours after initial dose.*

—OR—

For ampicillin/amoxicillin/penicillin-allergic patients unable to take oral medications:

Clindamycin 300 mg IV 30 minutes before a procedure and 150 mg IV (or orally) 6 hours after initial dose.*

B. For patients considered to be at high risk who are not candidates for the standard regimen:

Ampicillin 2.0 g IV (or IM) plus gentamicin 1.5 mg/kg IV (or IM) (not to exceed 80 mg) 30 minutes before procedure, followed by amoxicillin 1.5 g orally 6 hours after the initial dose. Alternatively, the parenteral regimen may be repeated 8 hours after the initial dose.*

For amoxicillin/ampicillin/penicillin-allergic patients considered to be at high risk:

Vancomycin 1.0 g IV administered over one hour, starting one hour before the procedure. No repeat dose is necessary.*

*Note: Initial pediatric dosages are listed below. Follow-up oral dose should be one-half the initial dose. Total pediatric dose should not exceed total adult dose.

Amoxicillin:†	50 mg/kg	Vancomycin:	20 mg/kg
Clindamycin:	10 mg/kg	Ampicillin:	50 mg/kg
Erythromycin ethylsuccinate		Gentamicin:	2.0 mg/kg
or stearate:	20 mg/kg		

†The following weight ranges may also be used for the initial pediatric dose of amoxicillin:

<15 kg (33 lbs), 750 mg
15-30 kg (33-66 lbs), 1500 mg
>30 kg (66 lbs), 3000 mg (full adult dose)

Kilogram to pound conversion chart: (1 kg = 2.2 lb)

Kg	Lb.
5	11.0
10	22.0
20	44.0
30	66.0
40	88.0
50	110.0

For Genitourinary/Gastrointestinal Procedures

I. Standard regimen:

Ampicillin 2.0 g IV (or IM) plus gentamicin 1.5 mg/kg IV (or IM) (not to exceed 80 mg) 30 minutes before procedure, followed by amoxicillin 1.5 g orally 6 hours after the initial dose. Alternatively, the parenteral regimen may be repeated once 8 hours after the initial dose.**

For amoxicillin/ampicillin/penicillin-allergic patients:

Vancomycin 1.0 g IV administered over 1 hour plus gentamicin 1.5 mg/kg IV (or IM) (not to exceed 80 mg) one hour before the procedure. May be repeated once 8 hours after initial dose.**

II. Alternate oral regimen for low-risk patients:

Amoxicillin 3.0 g orally one hour before the procedure, then 1.5 g 6 hours after the initial dose.**

Note: Initial pediatric dosages are listed below. Follow-up oral dose should be one-half the initial dose. Total pediatric dose should not exceed total adult dose.

Ampicillin:	50 mg/kg	Gentamicin:	2.0 mg/kg
Amoxicillin:	50 mg/kg	Vancomycin:	20 mg/kg

Note: Antibiotic regimens used to prevent recurrences of acute rheumatic fever are inadequate for the prevention of bacterial endocarditis. In patients with markedly compromised renal function, it may be necessary to modify or omit the second dose of gentamicin or vancomycin. Intramuscular injections may be contraindicated in patients receiving anticoagulants.

Adapted from *Prevention of Bacterial Endocarditis: Recommendations by the American Heart Association* by the Committee on Rheumatic Fever, Endocarditis, and Kawasaki Disease. JAMA 1990; 264-2919-2922. ©1990 American Medical Association (also excerpted in J Am Dent Assoc 1991;122:87-92).

Please refer to these joint American Heart Association - American Dental Association recommendations for more complete information as to which patients and which procedures require prophylaxis.

Reprinted courtesy of the American Heart Association.

- **Petechiae — Examination of the fundus with the ophthalmoscope may be helpful in detecting petechiae known as Roth spots, a sign of infective endocarditis. They can be multiple or single.**

When looking at the conjunctivae of the eyes, pull the lower lid downward so that the endothelial lining of the lid is better exposed. Occasionally a petechiae can be seen only when this maneuver is done. It is even better to grasp the lower lid between the index finger and thumb and then to pull the lower lid down, thereby "cupping" the lower lid; in this way one can see farther down and on occasion (personal experience) this has been the place the characteristic petechiae were found.

- **Emboli — Today, one does not often see the infected emboli that can occur with infective endocarditis. However, when they do occur they can be helpful in making the diagnosis of infective endocarditis.**

- **Splinter Hemorrhages** — **These signs of infective endocarditis may be found under the nails, often only if one searches for them.**

However, sometimes "pseudo-splinter" hemorrhages may be seen in people who do manual labor. In these people, without any other signs of infective endocarditis, these splinters are "red herrings".

- **Distinguishing between Janeway Lesions and Osler's Nodes** — **Janeway lesions are small, reddish, vascular lesions seen on the soles of the feet or the palms of the hands and are non-tender. Osler's Nodes are small, slightly raised, reddish areas seen on the tips of the toes or fingers and are tender.**

At times it is difficult to remember which of these lesions are the tender ones. I have an easy way of remembering: I knew Dr. Charles Janeway and he was a very nice man. He would not hurt anyone. I am sure Osler was too, but I never had the pleasure of meeting him.

Relative to infective endocarditis, staphylococcus infections of the skin (boils) can be the source of infective endocarditis, particularly in patients having valvular or congenital heart disease. Poorly recognized is the fact that shoes may be the culprit: Since many people put on their shoes before their pants, organisms such as staphylococci can be rubbed off and deposited in the cloth of the pants and subsequently in the pores and hair follicles. Therefore, when dressing: pants first, then shoes.

Dirty, infected shoes used to be brought to the operating rooms by surgeons (and other medical personnel) who kept their prize comfortable relics to wear during a surgical procedure. Cultures taken from these shoes were frequently positive. Fortunately sterile clean footwear is now used.

- **On Taking a History** — **When taking a history, ask your patient: "What have you been told about the diagnosis of your heart condition?"**

Surprisingly, in some, an accurate diagnosis is made by the patient, who knows specific details of his or her problem, including laboratory findings, results of diagnostic workup, and surgery if this had been performed. However, we should not cut short our own careful clinical evaluation because of this because the facts related by the patient can be incorrect and misleading.

At a teaching conference some years ago at Walter Reed Army Hospital, I was presented several "unknowns" for me to examine, diagnose and discuss. Examining the next to last patient, I placed both hands over the precordium and said:

- **"This is a cardiac pearl: if there is dextrocardia present (in a patient with a normal sized chest and not obese) we should not miss diagnosing this immediately, since we would feel the cardiac impulse on the right side instead of the left."**

This patient, however, did not have dextrocardia. As I said this, I noticed two physicians in the front row turn to each other and grin. (I wondered if they were smiling about a private joke or something and not paying attention to the patient's examination.)

The next — and last — patient had to be examined quickly, since the conference was just about to end. The patient was obese. She had symptoms consistent with mitral stenosis: shortness of breath on exertion and effort, such as making beds, vacuuming and/or scrubbing the floor, climbing stairs, etc. She even had what appeared to be a malar flush of mitral stenosis (a reddish coloration over the malar eminences of the face as if she used rouge or "blush").

On physical examination, I forgot to use both hands on palpating the chest, and I had difficulty in palpating the left ventricle, which I attributed to her significant obesity and very large breasts. On auscultation, I had difficulty in hearing the sounds. I was then told by the moderator of the conference to hurry up and conclude. It then dawned on me that they were playing a trick on me, and had presented a patient that had a history and physical appearance of mitral stenosis, but did not have it.

I was then asked: "Show us the diastolic rumble of mitral stenosis." I then replied: "I don't hear it." Then, I was asked, "Why don't you use both hands on palpation of this patient?" I then did so and you have guessed it — The cardiac impulse was on the *right* side, not the left and a classic diastolic rumble of mitral stenosis was present and heard by all (by means of multiple stethoscopes) — In the midst of continuing chuckles and laughter. No one attending that conference will ever forget this cardiac pearl, especially me. I don't think I have overlooked dextrocardia since that time.

Apropos to this was at a teaching conference several months ago at a university hospital in South Carolina. I was a visiting teacher and patients were presented as unknowns. I had previously mentioned the cardiac pearl of asking the patient about his or her diagnosis. A lady about 50 years of age was presented. I asked her: "What have you been told about your heart problem?" She immediately said: "I have dextrocardia" and she accurately described extra details of her problem. The physician conducting the conference had been at the Walter Reed Hospital conference just described, and he was hoping that I might forget to palpate with both hands. The "tables were turned" on my physician friend much to the enjoyment of the audience and especially myself. Two cardiac pearls were thereby emphasized.

- **At times, proper and efficient auscultation over the chest and neck is accomplished by having the patient stop breathing. In this way** breath sounds are not interfering. When we ask the patient to do so, we too, should also stop breathing. This reminds us when to tell the patient to resume breathing; if we don't remember, we may find our patient struggling to keep from taking a breath.

- **When listening over the supraclavicular area and neck, it is absolutely necessary to have the patient stop breathing because of the distraction of the loud breath sounds.**

Sometimes a particularly garrulous patient continues to talk while we try to listen; several things are helpful: (a) politely ask to please stop talking, (b) say: "Let me see your tongue," (c) "Hold your breath." Along these lines and pertaining to some of our fellow men and women: one of the most common of the tachycardias and often the hardest to treat, is "mandibular tachycardia;" some even have "mandibular fibrillation." Sometimes, I, too, am guilty of this when giving a lecture; I state this showing this final slide (Figure 82).

It is my impression that lawyers give the most accurately detailed account of their history. Sometimes when I do not know an occupation of a particular patient and he states: "On July 19, at 1:00 PM I was walking on the left side of Main Street, I noticed etc." I then ask: "By the way, are you an attorney": and the answer is "Yes". Have you noticed this too?

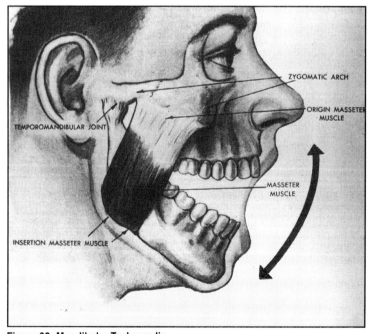

Figure 82: Mandibular Tachycardia

More Miscellaneous

It is wise to screen carefully for evidence of cardiac decompensation in patients who are to have surgery. As discussed previously (page 1) the detection of pulsus alternans, alternation of the intensity of the second sound, and murmurs provide clues. If present and not diagnosed previously, then treatment can be instituted and surgery can be delayed for several days. This is especially apropos for elderly patients with known or unknown cardiac decompensation. Taking extra days to make sure there is optimal medical control of the problem can be prophylactic against complications with surgery. For example, many patients have extra edema fluid which can be removed with a mild diuretic. A word of caution, however, regarding use of a diuretic and loss of a significant amount of fluid. I recall reports of patients who had a stroke coincident with the surgery, and in whom dehydration with the diuretic was thought to be a contributing factor. Therefore delay surgery for several days.

- **An electrocardiogram pre and postoperatively should be routine, as a myocardial infarction can occur during surgery and be "silent" because of the anesthesia.**

- **Physical Activity — "Do what you can do *in comfort*. Avoid extremes of exertion in extremes of weather."**

    I call this my "old fashioned rule". The very bitter cold weather is the worst and next is hot, humid weather. This rule has evolved over the years as a valuable cardiac pearl and has "stood the test of time." It will answer many questions that arise in the minds of cardiac patients. For example, if a patient wonders whether he should climb several flights of stairs or walk up a certain incline, I tell him that if he can do so without any symptoms or discomfort, then it is fine. This rule is applicable to a wide range of physical activities and enables patients to judge for themselves whether that particular activity is causing any untoward symptoms for them. This also applies to sexual intercourse.

- **Sexual intercourse should be discussed freely with the patient who has heart disease.**

    Too often, the patient and spouse are reluctant to bring this up for discussion and they appreciate the physician initiating it. Most patients can resume sexual intercourse several weeks to several months after returning home following an acute myocardial infarction, or after treatment for other cardiac problems, including cardiac surgery. Again, remember the old fashioned rule, "do what you can do in comfort, avoiding extremes of exertion in extremes of weather."

Not uncommonly, patients having coronary bypass surgery or repair of a valvular lesion may ask whether their hemorrhoids or hernia could be repaired at the same time. The answer is "No." It is better to do the major surgery alone, and then subsequently have the other surgery if there are enough symptoms to warrant it.

- **Questions About Anesthesia — Cardiac patients often ask, "What anesthetic should I have?" The answer is, of course, that you choose the surgeon and let him and the anesthesiologist choose the anesthesia.**

- **Choosing a Surgeon — If a patient needs coronary bypass surgery or valve replacement, what is your advice concerning the selection of the surgeon? Ask yourself what surgeon you would have for a member of your own family or yourself.**

Your answer to this question is the surgeon to recommend for your patient. Even if that particular surgeon is in another institution in another city, this advice still holds.

- **Timing of Surgery — Patients frequently ask, "If I will need cardiac surgery some time in the future, why not do it now?" The same question may be asked by a referring physician. For the patient who is asymptomatic and leading an essentially normal life, it is wise to be conservative.**

Follow the patient closely at regular intervals, and advise surgery when significant signs and symptoms become evident. One may be pleasantly surprised (the patient as well as the physician) by the length of time that may pass before a decision for surgery has to be made. There are also a number of such patients that live a normal life span and *never* have to face the surgery.

The buying of time frequently pays off. The mortality from surgical procedures usually becomes progressively lower with the passage of time, due to improvement in surgical techniques and postoperative care. Therefore, be conservative in the asymptomatic patient, but on the other hand be prepared to move quickly with any significant change in status.

I have had the responsibility to recommend both cardiac and non-cardiac surgery for a large number of patients having heart disease. Over the period of time, I was impressed how often patients — probably about 25% — (who came from all sections of our country) had been given a prognosis as to how long they could live because of their heart disease. What became evident was that the prediction was often grossly wrong and sometimes the patient outlived the doctor.

- **Don't be a prophet! It is better to tell the patient and/or members of the family that no one can usually accurately prognosticate and to think positively rather than negatively: "Let's talk about living — not dying."**

I have found it unwise to quote statistics when answering the question; "Doctor, what are my chances of surviving the operation?" This simple answer usually suffices: "The risk of having the surgery is less than not having it;" or when appropriate, to say: "there is always some risk of surgery, but in your case it is low."

The great majority of patients and their families are satisfied and often relieved with this answer.

I have found that when numbers concerning mortality are cited, undue fears and anxiety can result; helpful to counteract this: "You are not a *number,* a *statistic.* You are an individual and will be treated as such."

Acceptance of surgery by the patient and family is, of course, a disturbing and sometimes difficult decision. Unless there is great urgency or an emergency, I have found worthwhile this important cardiac pearl — the "trial period:"

- **"Why don't we have a trial period of 3 to 6 months (which might include a new medication or an even tighter medical regimen); if you are no worse, or better, then we can have another trial period."**

If, however, at the end of the trial period the patient is worse, then everyone (patient, physician and family) accepts the reality that operation is necessary and that strict medical management cannot suffice.

Also good advice that helps the patient realize it has to be done: "You need the operation. Don't put it off; you will only 'stew' and agonize over it, so go ahead and get it over with."

As we physicians know, a long delay can result in further deterioration of the patient's physical condition making surgery even more risky; unfortunately, even death can occur. Once the decision for surgery is accepted it is helpful and reassuring for the patient to meet not only the surgeon, but other members of the surgical team including the anesthesiologist.

- **A Preoperative Cardiac Pearl: "When you return from the operating room and** wake up, you will have tubes: from your mouth for assistance in breathing and ventilation, nose for oxygen, chest for drainage, intravenous fluid, etc; you will be surrounded by elaborate and sophisticated equipment plus trained personnel who are looking after you. Do not be alarmed and think something is wrong. Remember, this is normal and is why things go well in the recovery period."

I have had many patients tell me: "I am so glad that you told me what to expect; otherwise I would have thought that there were serious complications and I might die." Too often, the patient's spouse or family has not been told of what to expect in the pre and postoperative periods. Unnecessary fears, anxieties and misunderstanding with resentment result. Putting ourselves in the place of patients and/or their families will remind us and insure that we talk, explain and reassure them; also letting them know we care. These simple things which we and the staff can provide should not be absent in any hospital.

"You have a problem with your heart, but you would be an unusual patient if you cannot be helped." This is certainly true of the great majority of patients we see with cardiovascular disease. Whether in the hospital or office, a patient being evaluated for the first time should have this encouragement as an initial and integral part of treatment. All we have to do is to put ourselves in the patient's place to realize how important this is.

- **"Week-End Athlete" — Don't be a "week-end", "monthly", or "yearly" athlete, particularly if you are in middle age or older.**

Serious consequences may result — arrhythmias, myocardial infarction, dizziness, syncope or near syncope. An example: A man in his fifties was raking leaves in his yard. He suddenly recalled his athlete years on the track team in college. Having heard so much about how exercise is good for us, he dropped his rake and set out: first walking at a fast rate, then a faster pace and finally sprinting. He collapsed; he had produced a complete heart block which was permanent. One wonders when, if ever, this would have occurred if he had not succumbed to that impulse to race as he did on the track team in college.

- **Walking is an excellent form of exercise that one can do throughout all of life (no likelihood of joint problems, of pain and traumatic arthritis, bone spurs, etc. that can result from other types of exercise such as jogging).**

About 20 years ago, a friend and colleague who is a cardiologist and exercise physiologist related to me that he had just completed some studies comparing walking and jogging. He found that if you walk *several* miles per day *several* days a week, you keep a conditioning similar to that from jogging. The walk should be more "on the brisk side" than "ambling". Take your walks on days of good weather.

- **The Five Year Rule — We have a "five year rule": A new drug, procedure, technique or piece of equipment should ideally stand the test of time — about five years — before it is fully utilized.**

    If at the end of this "watching" period nothing negative has evolved, then it may be utilized as indicated. If, on the other hand, there are complications or side effects, they usually become evident within the five year time span. An example: Some years ago, a certain antihypertensive drug was being advocated at a symposium. I was asked, "Are you using this drug?" I answered, "I am aware of it and watching it, but it has not yet passed my five year rule." I said that I had heard of a couple of patients who developed cataracts while on the medication and also knew of several patients who complained of their hair falling out (losing an excessive amount of hair when combing). I pointed out that each of these complications might well be coincidence, but more time was needed to evaluate this new drug. A year later these complications of the drug were established and it was taken off the market. Of course, many patients have urgent need for a new drug or procedure which should be utilized for the best and proper treatment under the circumstances.

- **How to enjoy an egg, yet minimize cholesterol.**

    I have seen many patients who bemoan the fact that they can no longer have eggs for breakfast, since they are on a low fat, low cholesterol diet. I, too, enjoy an egg for breakfast and for many years have used the following expedient:

    For a fried egg, I use a frying pan with a teflon-type of coating and for my "medium" cooked egg, turn it over; the yolk (which is 100% cholesterol) is then broken with the spatula, expressed out and discarded (or given to a happy dog). A small amount of the yolk is left but, like garlic, provides some flavor to the egg white, which is a good source of protein.

    For a boiled egg, which I also like, after about six minutes of boiling I remove the egg, crack it open and discard all but a little bit of yolk which, as in the case of the fried egg, provides some flavor to the white.

    Many of my patients have tried these "cardiac (egg) pearls" for breakfast and say, "Now I enjoy breakfast again."

- **Diet — Adherence is important, but exceptions can be made for special occasions.**

The majority of our patients are conscientious about following advice concerning diets (sodium restricted, low fat-low cholesterol, diabetic, etc.). However, I have found that some have the impression that even a single non-adherence meal might have some dire effect. We tell our patients that careful adherence to their diet is necessary, but not to make a fetish of it, and on occasions such as eating out at a good restaurant or at a banquet where their usual diet is not possible, to enjoy it, and resume their diet with the next meal.

When patients who are on a strict sodium diet have a non-diet meal they may retain large amounts of fluid. These patients are advised to take an extra diuretic pill when they return home, thereby anticipating and counteracting the extra fluid retention.

● Ascorbic acid on fish to make it flavor like salt.

For those on a low salt diet, use a small amount of ascorbic acid on fish instead of salt; this can fool the taste buds to think it is salt. (A tablet of ascorbic acid can be crushed or scraped into a powder, but be sure to use only a small amount, otherwise the taste will be unpleasant. I recently learned this cardiac pearl from Dr. Marshall Franklin of Scripps Clinic, San Diego.)

Restriction of sodium in the diet is one of the most important aspects in treatment of congestive heart failure. The patient should be advised, and become knowledgeable, concerning the sodium content of various foods and drinks.

Concerning sodium intake, a number of people still use baking soda to clean their teeth. After brushing with baking soda and rinsing the mouth with water, residual soda can remain and thereby be swallowed. Therefore, patients having cardiac decompensation should be advised against the use of baking soda as a dentifrice.

● Recently, baking soda has been added to some of the pastes or gels. I have tried this, and find that I still taste the baking soda even after rinsing.

Gargling with baking soda added to heated water as a treatment for sore throat (or as a mouthwash) has been used for decades; although a less common practice today, it is still utilized by some. Sodium is absorbed from this procedure and therefore patients having to restrict sodium in their diet should refrain.

● Bone Tired Fatigue

I have been impressed with the following scenario that may lead to an acute heart attack.

First the patient is "bone tired" — this is more than the usual fatigue that is so common with everyone. It is an extreme type of fatigue. The patient lives on the east coast (e.g., Washington, D.C.). He has a special important presentation or commitment on the west coast. Contributing to this undue fatigue, he has worked long hours preparing for his trip. He has lost sleep. He smokes cigarettes too much, eats poorly. Finally he makes his trip. He lands on the west coast (San Francisco) at 10:00 PM his time. It is 7:00 PM San Francisco time. He is met by his hosts who take him out to dinner where more than his usual cocktail and food are consumed. Being a businessman, he is under increased stress and tension to promote his products. He is brought back to his hotel at midnight west coast time which is 3:00 in the morning (his eastern time). What little sleep he gets is restless; he wakes up at 7:00 AM his time (4:00 AM California time) and can't go back to sleep. He therefore had only several hours sleep.

During the day he continues under unusual stress trying to complete his business deal or mission. He has "jet lag" — a *real* thing! He then repeats the sequence of events the next evening and night and perhaps another day and night. He is unusually fatigued and definitely "bone tired." An acute myocardial infarction may now occur.

I have observed this scenario on repeated occasions and am convinced that this can often lead to an acute myocardial infarction.

It is apparent that this unusual extreme fatigue should be avoided. Try to stay on your own "time" as much as possible. Extra rest and sleep should take place before getting into the situation as just described. The patient, his wife, and family can be alerted to always avoid it if possible.

My wife at times has reminded me, "You know when you talk about being fatigued and "bone tired"? That's the way you are now." I try to pay attention to her observations; then I try to break the cycle and get extra rest and sleep over the next several days.

Some Cardiac Pearl
Answers to Patients' Questions

Q. What is meant by angina pectoris?

A. Angina means pain. Pectoris means chest. Therefore "chest pain". Ingrained in our vocabulary today, however, is the connotation implying correctly, of course, that this is the pain associated with coronary artery disease and/or heart muscle (lack of or decreased oxygen to the heart muscle, which is termed "ischemia").

Q. I keep my nitroglycerin tablets in my nice metal pill box. A friend of mine told me I should use a glass container. Is this true?

A. Yes. There is much less chance of deterioration of the potency of the nitroglycerin tablets if they are kept in glass. Avoid metal or plastic boxes or aluminum "strip" type of packaging. Nitroglycerin tablets can deteriorate in weeks to months in these containers. As you know, some of the medicine pill boxes are fancy and expensive, made of silver, gold and even embroidered at times with jewels. So, I have to reluctantly tell my patients to stay with the small glass bottle in which they are generally dispensed.

Q. Is there any way I can tell when my nitroglycerin tablets have lost their strength?

A. The nitroglycerin tablet taken sublingually (under the tongue) will usually have a "sting" or produce a slight burning sensation. Also, if the side effect of "fullness of the head," flushing, or some headache took place, these would also indicate that the tablet is working. The tablet of nitroglycerin which is not effective in relieving the chest discomfort of angina but had always worked, should be a clue that the medication could be too old, although of course, it could represent a new change of more obstruction in the coronary vessels. Be sure to call this to your doctor's attention.

Q. I have heart trouble and have to take a daily diuretic to eliminate the extra fluid. I have been told to eat foods that have a high content of potassium. Why? What are the best foods to eat that have a higher content of potassium?

A. The sodium of sodium chloride — salt, NaCl — present in our body tissues holds water similar to a sponge. The diuretic causes excretion of sodium, which in turn pulls the extra fluid (water) that has accumulated. Most effective diuretics also cause excretion of potassium. You need to replace the potassium that has been eliminated and sometimes this can be done by eating fruits and vegetables that have a good potassium content. A list supplied by the American Heart Association appears on page 16.

At times your physician will prescribe supplemental potassium to take in the form of tablets, capsules or liquids to insure that potassium levels of blood are properly maintained. The symptoms of low potassium are listed on page 16.

Q. My doctor diagnosed my heart condition as heart failure. Does this mean there is now no hope for me?

A. The use of the term "heart failure" is an unfortunate one because it can cause undue anxiety in patients. The term cardiac decompensation would be a better one and there are varying degrees of decompensation. At times it is very mild, other times of a moderate degree, other times of a more severe degree. Prompt recognition of the early signs of cardiac decompensation will lead to the institution of the proper medication and diet and advice as to the proper type of physical activity. Today, we are fortunate in having excellent medications that are aimed at the control of cardiac decompensation. Also, it is important that your physician determine the reason why your heart has become less efficient than normal. At times, this is completely correctable and at other times methods of treatment can be instituted on a long-term basis that can enable the patient to continue leading a comfortable type of life.

Q. My husband is taking an anticoagulant called "coumadin". I have heard that other drugs can enhance its action and bleeding can result. Is this true?

A. Yes. Aspirin is one of these. A list of drugs causing interaction with coumadin (as well as with other drugs) is available and often is distributed by local pharmacists if requested. It is important that the patient and other responsible members of the family become aware of the interaction of the drugs that are prescribed.

Q. I have been told by my physician that I have left bundle branch block. I am now afraid that this means there is blockage of blood in the heart. How dangerous is this? Am I prone to "sudden death"?

A. The term "bundle branch block", which may be either left or right, is an unfortunate one in many respects. It is an electrical phenomenon in the heart and has nothing to do with the actual blockage of blood; instead, it indicates that the electrical impulse is blocked. Illustrating this was a nursing instructor about 55 years of age. I first examined her approximately six years before. At that time she had hypertension for which she was treated, with satisfactory control of her blood pressure. I was asked to now evaluate her again and when I took her history, I read a report from her physician stating that she now showed left bundle branch block on her electrocardiogram. I then said to her, "I think I may know what is bothering you, in that you now think that you have blockage of blood in your heart from circulation." She said, "Yes." When I explained to her that this was not the case she proclaimed, "Thank God! I have been worried sick for the past months thinking I might get a complete blockage of the heart and then I would die suddenly." Her treatment: Merely understanding that bundle branch block does not mean blockage of blood. It does not necessarily mean that some dire event is bound to happen. In fact, there are many patients that have left bundle branch block for many, many years without any symptoms whatsoever. However, this can be evaluated and explained to the patient by a physician. As a rule, the outlook can be good as far as this specific finding is concerned. Right bundle branch block carries an even better outlook, if this is the only finding, and can be present for many years without any symptoms whatsoever.

People are living longer today — All one has to do is read the obituary columns of our newspapers and note the ages of death. The majority of these are in their 70s, 80s and even 90s.

When the age of death is in the 30s or 40s, there is often a statement: "He had AIDS." This frightening disease is unquestionably increasing at an alarming rate. Deaths in the 40s, 50s, and early 60s are often related to cancer.

If we checked the ages at death several decades ago, the average seemed to be 10 years or more less than it is at present. There are a number of factors responsible for this: Better medicines and treatment of heart disease; preventive measures including: stopping smoking of cigarettes and other uses of tobacco, detection and control of diabetes, better diet and control of cholesterol.

The public is now aware of risk factors of coronary disease. Anyone who shops in the grocery store is almost overwhelmed by the advertising and labels on items of food stating, "low cholesterol," "zero cholesterol," "low fat," "low calories," etc. Many of our patients know the recommended levels of blood lipid determinations of cholesterol, HDL, LDL, HDL/LDL. This would have been almost unheard of 10 years (or more) ago. Coronary disease has had a significant reduction in morbidity and mortality.

Hypertension

- **Control of hypertension — This has been an important factor in the increase in longevity.**

    This is due not only to better detection of hypertension, but also to treatment and follow up to make sure that there is compliance and especially the proper and effective medication being used.

    Stroke is a frequent "end of the road" complication of hypertension. This can often be prevented by adequate management of hypertension for which we now have excellent drugs for treatment.

    Worthy of emphasis: Detect hypertension early, treat early, avoid stroke, live longer.

- **Should we treat systolic hypertension when the diastolic pressure is normal? Yes. This is now well established, whereas in the not too distant past it was believed that this was not necessary.**

    It is not unusual today to evaluate patients in the eighth decade of age or older who are overly concerned about eating fats and cholesterol in their diet. I frequently tell them to eat what they want and not to worry about it.

    Some patients with coronary artery disease have angina after eating a large meal; others have angina after a heavy meal plus walking up an incline in cold weather. Eating smaller, more frequent meals can be of help in some patients.

    Stay thin — live longer. Most patients who are very obese do not live to the ripe old age of 80 and above. Those who do are usually thin.

    I once asked this question to the entire senior class of our medical school: "How many of you have ever seen a very fat old man?" At first there was no answer and then one student said: "Winston Churchill." Of course this great English leader in World War II was known to have several risk factors of coronary heart disease including smoking, poor diet, alcohol use, and stress. He obviously was an exception to the rule. Perhaps his inherited genes were an important factor in this respect.

- **Most older people do not eat as much as when they were younger. Many also begin to eat** more sweets. This "sweet tooth" tendency is not a good thing for those predisposed to late onset diabetes. Remember, obesity predisposes to hypertension, diabetes and coronary disease.

- **Poorly recognized facts:** (a) The obese person who has hypertension may be pleasantly surprised to find that a loss of 30 pounds of weight often can reduce the blood pressure to normal levels. (b) Loss of weight plus diet can also control diabetes (particularly late onset type), thereby avoiding medication.

Patients having chronic heart disease with cardiac decompensation are frequently thin. They lose muscle tissue weight prompting them to say: "I have lost weight and I don't like looking this thin." It can be explained to them that this is a frequent occurrence and not to worry about it.

- **To illustrate to an obese patient who may complain of shortness of breath, I have weighed different objects in the office or examining room such as a chair or a piece of medical apparatus. For example, I had an ECG machine in the examining room that weighed about 30 pounds. I would say: "Lift up that machine." The patient doing so might remark, "Oh, that's heavy." Then I say "You are constantly carrying one (or two) ECG machines. No wonder you are short of breath." This is especially pertinent to the patient with heart disease, emphasizing why excess weight is not desirable.**

Alcohol and the Heart

The use of alcohol frequently results in heart problems:

- **Alcoholic Cardiomyopathy — Consumption of alcohol in large quantities over a long period of time (years) unquestionably can cause cardiomyopathy of the dilated type. (See discussion of Dilated Cardiomyopathy, Gallop Rhythm and Congestive Heart Failure)**

The heart muscle is affected, producing symptoms and signs of heart failure and arrhythmias. Sudden death can occur in addition to death from chronic advanced cardiac decompensation.

If determined early enough, reversal of the problem can occur via early treatment, including *total abstinence* from alcohol (which is often difficult). "Hard liquor" as well as beer and wine consumption can lead to alcoholic cardiomyopathy.

Alcohol in smaller amounts, such as several cocktails or glasses of wine, can "trigger" (or precipitate) arrhythmias in the patient who has underlying heart disease. This occurs much more frequently than is generally realized; premature beats and atrial fibrillation can occur causing uncomfortable symptoms in the patient. At times, atrial fibrillation with a rapid ventricular rate produces cardiac decompensation — even pulmonary edema. If a careful history elicits a recurrent arrhythmia such as atrial fibrillation following even small amounts of alcohol ingestion, it is wise to advise our patient to refrain from its use. However, some patients do not heed such advice and have the recurrent problem; as a prophylaxis in such reluctant patients, an antiarrhythmic pill such as quinidine taken before alcohol ingestion can sometimes be used with success. Fortunately, however, the majority follow the advice of *no alcohol*.

Alcohol, usually in larger amounts, or "binges" can produce arrhythmias such as atrial fibrillation in a perfectly normal heart. I recall seeing a young sailor at a teaching conference in a naval hospital, who after a weekend "binge" had atrial fibrillation which required hospitalization; the electrocardiogram documented atrial fibrillation. After reversion to normal sinus rhythm, the "p" waves in the limb leads and in lead V_1 indicated left atrial enlargement; these were transient changes. In addition, transient left atrial enlargement was also demonstrated on the heart x-rays.

From a clinical point of view, it is probable that ingestion of a large amount of alcohol in a patient with heart disease (such as coronary artery disease or cardiomyopathy) can "trigger" a ventricular arrhythmia causing sudden death.

Innocent Systolic Murmurs

- ***The innocent systolic murmur* is short, occurring in early to mid systole. It is not holosystolic. Normal splitting of the second heart sound is present also (Figure 83).**

One of the more frequent reasons why a patient is referred to a physician is the evaluation of a systolic murmur. The innocent murmur can be diagnosed in the physician's office or at the bedside. This is accomplished by using the so-called "five finger" approach (See figure on page XIII). This entails a total clinical cardiovascular

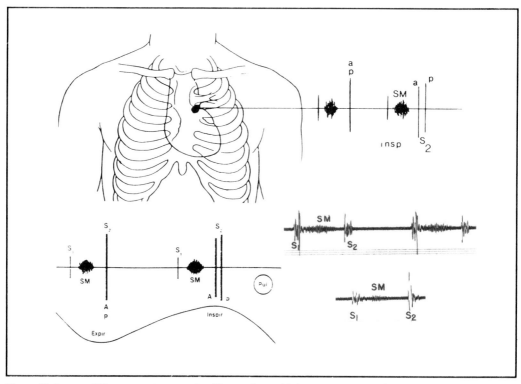

Figure 83: Innocent Murmurs – A composite of four patients with innocent murmurs (SM). The murmur is short in duration and occurs in early to mid-systole. Note normal splitting of the second sound (S_2, A-P), single with expiration (expir) and widening with inspiration (insp), shown in top and lower left panels.

evaluation, including a detailed history and physical examination, the electrocardiogram, the chest x-ray, and more simple, appropriate laboratory tests. These five fingers can clench and make a fist, and this gives a very powerful, efficient way of making a clinical diagnosis, without the necessity of more elaborate procedures that can be performed only in a hospital setting.

The innocent systolic murmur is very common. It is a frequent finding in children and teenagers, and less likely in adults. On one occasion I had the opportunity to carefully search for the presence of a murmur in approximately 100 school children, average age 11 or 12. I found approximately 60% who had an innocent systolic murmur. It is also of interest that in this particular group I found 100% had a normal physiologic third heart sound; 100% had a normal physiologic venous hum that was detected listening over the right supraclavicular fossa, with the head turned "on a stretch" to the opposite direction (Figure 84). Short systolic murmurs (bruits) were noted in both the right and left supraclavicular fossae in about 25 or 30% (Figure 85). The innocent systolic murmur is early to mid systolic (Figure 86); it is generally grade 1 to 3 on a basis of six (Samuel A. Levine's classification); splitting of the second

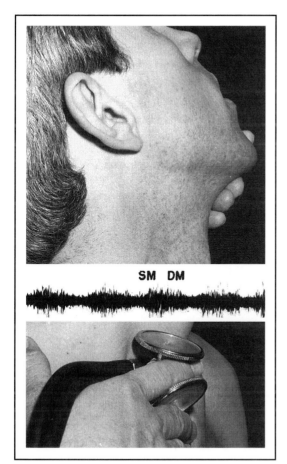

SM DM

Figure 84: To Detect a Venous Hum: Listening with the bell of the stethoscope over the right supraclavicular fossa, the physician's left hand moves the patient's head to the opposite direction (left) and "on a stretch."

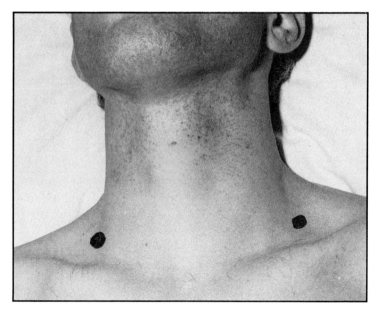

Figure 85: Right and Left Supraclavicular Fossae — Innocent short, early to mid-systolic murmurs can be heard over these areas.

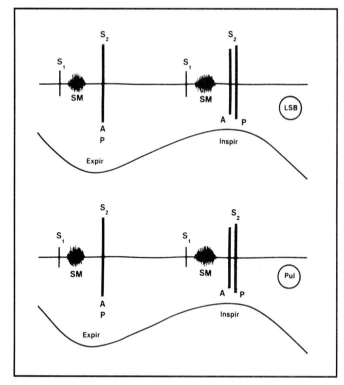

Figure 86: Innocent early to mid systolic murmur (SM) and normal splitting (A-P) of the second sound (S₂).

heart sound is normal, becoming wider with inspiration and single or closely split with expiration. The electrocardiogram and cardiac silhouette of the heart are normal. The history is negative, except for the finding of a murmur.

- **Murmurs of pathologic conditions can be similar to innocent murmurs, but they have other associated findings. For example, atrial septal defect has wide, so-called "fixed" splitting of the second heart sound. The electrocardiogram has changes, particularly in lead V_1: right ventricular conduction delay (RSR_1), right bundle branch block or right ventricular hypertrophy. The x-ray shows increased blood flow in the lungs and enlarged pulmonary arteries.**

On auscultation, the innocent systolic murmur is similar, except there is a wide, so-called "fixed splitting" of the second sound with atrial defect.

The murmur of a congenital bicuspid aortic valve can in itself be similar to the innocent murmur, but an ejection sound is present with the aortic stenosis which is well heard over the precordium from the aortic area to the apex.

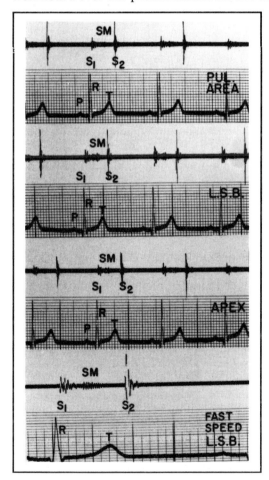

Figure 87: Innocent Murmur — The innocent systolic murmur (SM) is in early to mid systole and is heard over the various areas of the precordium, best in this patient at mid left sternal border (L.S.B.)

- **Location: A common misconception is that an innocent murmur is localized over one area, such as the pulmonic area, third left sternal border, or aortic area.**

  Instead, innocent murmurs are frequently heard in other areas of the precordium, although they may be loudest over one particular area (Figure 87). When such a murmur is present in one area, listen carefully over other areas and you usually will detect the same murmur, but it will be fainter. Sometimes the innocent murmur may be loudest at the apex; other times it may be louder over the pulmonic area.

- **Innocent systolic murmurs are commonly found in children and in the early teen years. They are less common in adults.**

  An interesting exception is the fact that innocent systolic murmurs were found in more than 90% of 90 National Football League players personally examined (Figures 88, 89).

  As mentioned, innocent systolic murmurs occur in early to mid-systole. They are generally Grade 1-3 in intensity and in the great majority are readily diagnosed in the office or at the bedside. The second heart sound is of normal intensity, normally split and the degree of splitting increases in normal fashion with inspiration. The total cardiovascular evaluation of these patients is normal (Figures 90, 91).

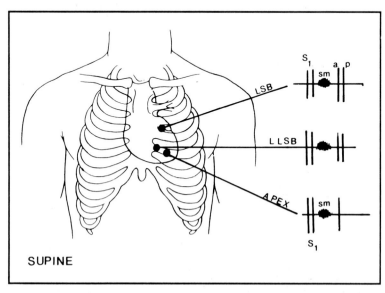

Figure 88: Football Player — The patient is an all-Pro NFL football player lying supine. Note wide split of first sound (S_1), innocent systolic murmur (sm), and wide split of S_2 (a-p) which became single on expiration in the sitting position.

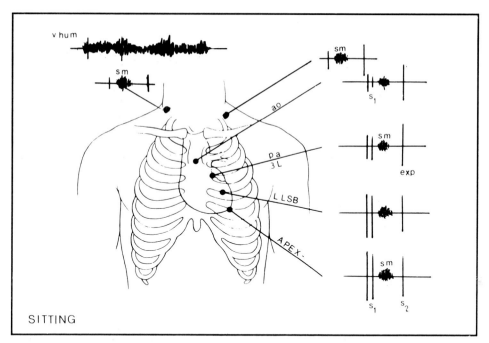

Figure 89: Same Patient — Sitting. S_2 becomes single with expiration (exp). Note innocent systolic murmur (sm) heard from apex to aortic area. On auscultation of the neck, note the short innocent systolic murmur (sm) at both the left and right supraclavicular areas. There is also a venous hum.

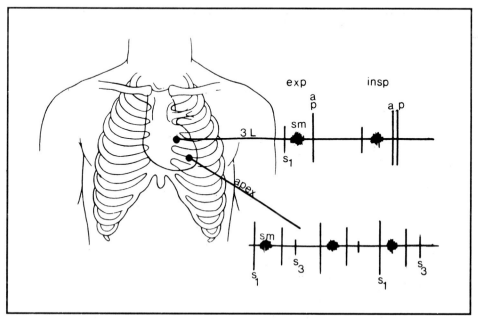

Figure 90: A 13-year old boy with normal splitting of the second sound (A-P) — wider on inspiration (insp). at 3L (3rd left sternal border). The normal third sound (S_3) waxes and wanes with respiration (apex). Note innocent systolic murmur (SM) at the apex and third left sternal border.

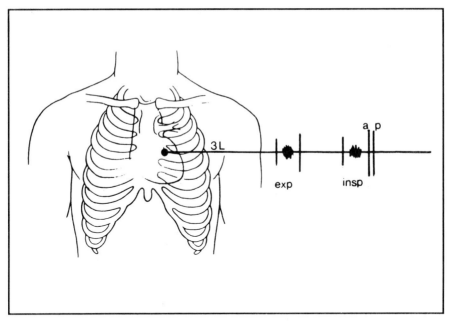

Figure 91: A 21-year old man with grade 2-3 innocent systolic murmur (SM). Normal splitting of second sound (A-P). Aortic (A) and pulmonic components of S$_2$ widen with inspiration (insp).

More sophisticated laboratory studies such as echocardiography and cardiac catheterization are usually not necessary for diagnosis and only add to the expense incurred by the patient or family.

• Differentiation from Other Conditions: Innocent systolic murmurs are often similar to murmurs caused by a bicuspid aortic valve, mild pulmonic stenosis, or atrial septal defect. How to tell the difference? Consider the concomitant findings (Figure 92):

1. A murmur due to a bicuspid aortic valve has an aortic ejection sound that is unaffected by respiration.

2. A murmur due to congenital valvular pulmonic stenosis also has an ejection sound but it will vary, becoming fainter or even disappearing on inspiration, although heard louder on expiration. The murmur of pulmonic stenosis also is more likely to have a wider split of the second heart sound that does not become single on expiration. Right ventricular hypertrophy may be noted on the electrocardiogram.

3. With a murmur due to atrial septal defect, there is wide "fixed" splitting of the second heart sound. This finding, together with the electrocardiographic and x-ray changes of atrial septal defect, can quickly make the distinction between this serious murmur and an innocent murmur.

Innocent murmurs are better heard in young people who have thin chests than in those who are obese or muscular.

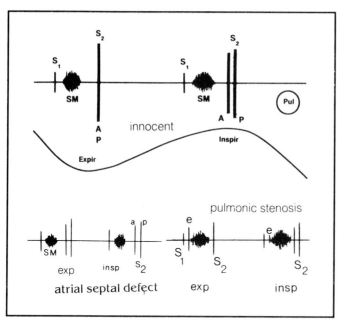

Figure 92: Comparisons: (Top) A patient with an innocent systolic murmur (SM). The second sound (S₂) is single with expiration (expir) and widens with inspiration (inspir). Lower left: Atrial septal defect. The systolic murmur (SM) is similar to the innocent, but there is wide splitting of the second sound with both expiration and inspiration. Lower right: Congenital valvular pulmonic stenosis. The systolic murmur is similar to the innocent, but there is an ejection sound (e) which gets fainter with inspiration.

- **Once the diagnosis of innocent murmur is established, it is not wise or necessary to have the patient return at intervals of several months or a year to keep check on this murmur. Otherwise it can be logically interpreted: "The doctor is not sure; if not, why do I have to return?"**

Reassure the patient and the parents (if he/she is a young person) that the murmur is innocent and explain how it is produced. As part of the reassurance I tell the patients that follow up visits are not necessary.

Recalled is a patient whom I saw in the office and made the diagnosis of an innocent systolic murmur. This was told to the patient. The patient then asked, "If my murmur is *innocent,* are the other murmurs *guilty*?" When you think about it that's not a bad term and deserves using, but of course the other murmurs are generally called "significant".

- **Systolic Murmur in the Elderly: Systolic murmurs in the elderly population are an expected and usually innocent finding.**

Since people are living longer today, this murmur will be detected even more often if it is searched for. It is usually grade 1 to 3 in intensity and best heard over the aortic area or left sternal border; it may also be heard over the clavicles (bone transmission), in the suprasternal notch, supraclavicular areas of the neck, including over the carotid arteries.

The murmur frequently has a somewhat musical quality and can be transmitted down to the apex (Figure 93). Sometimes it can even be better heard at the apex. Occasionally a faint aortic diastolic murmur (grade 1 or 2) is heard in addition to the systolic murmur. If the patient is asymptomatic and the electrocardiogram and chest x-ray reveal no significant findings related to aortic valve disease, then no further diagnostic studies are needed at that time.

An aortic ejection sound is not a feature of aortic stenosis of the elderly as it is with the congenital bicuspid aortic valve. The murmur has been described as the "innocent murmur of the elderly" and is related to some minimal sclerosis or other alteration of the aortic valve; some of these patients have varying amounts of calcium in the valve leaflets, but the commissures are not fibrosed and fused, and the valve functions well. While many such patients remain stable for a number of years, others progress to more extensive fibrosis, calcium deposits, and stenosis of the valve leaflets, thereby resulting in significant signs and symptoms necessitating valve replacement.

There are many types of systolic murmurs (Figure 94). It is useful to note the auscultatory interpretation of the configuration of these systolic murmurs. By paying attention to the specific portions of systole that the murmur occupies, this configuration can be readily detected by one's own stethoscope.

Sketch the configuration of the murmur as well as the components of the heart sounds and extra sounds, such as gallops, clicks, and ejection sounds (Figure 95). This

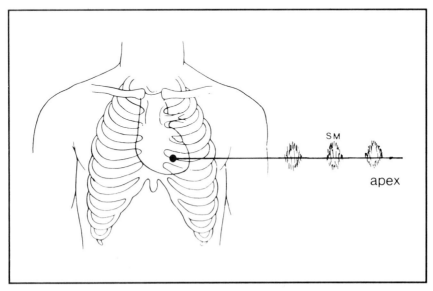

Figure 93: An elderly patient with emphysema having increased AP diameter of the chest. A high frequency, musical systolic murmur (SM) is heard, mainly at the apex. It is important to rule out aortic stenosis in such a patient.

is not difficult to do and it can be extremely helpful in diagnosis, as well as in developing one's own individual expertise. It is suggested that you sketch the auscultatory findings and put them in your own records as well as in the hospital records.

- **Cardiac Pearl:** **The person who carefully sketches what is heard on auscultation becomes progressively more expert in the art of auscultation. I have never seen an exception.**

- **Loud Murmurs That Can Be Heard Without a Stethoscope — Some very loud murmurs can be heard without a stethoscope, sometimes even several feet away from**

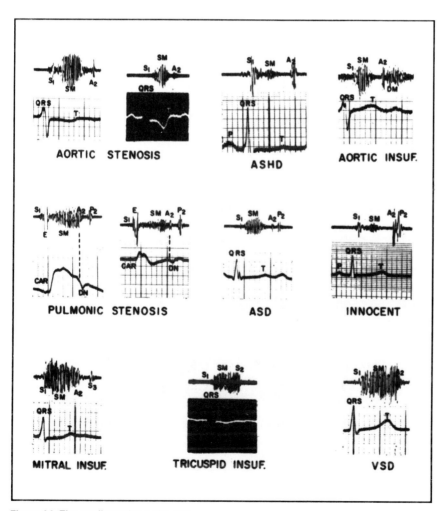

Figure 94: The configurations of systolic murmurs.

the patient. Conditions most likely to cause such a murmur are mitral valve prolapse, tricuspid valve prolapse, tricuspid regurgitation, or malfunction of a prosthetic valve.

Less likely causes are the loudest murmurs of aortic stenosis and pulmonic stenosis, traumatic arteriovenous fistula from shrapnel or bullet wounds or from automobile or airplane accidents, or traumatic rupture of a heart valve.

I recall one soldier who had an arteriovenous fistula due to a shrapnel wound. It produced a loud continuous murmur over his posterior chest. When he recovered consciousness after the injury, he thought the enemy tanks were coming because of the vibration due to his fistula while he was lying on the ground.

Another patient I remember was kicked in the chest by a horse. On recovery, he likened the sound emanating from his chest to that of a water pump on the farm where he grew up. He had traumatic rupture of his aortic valve, producing severe aortic regurgitation.

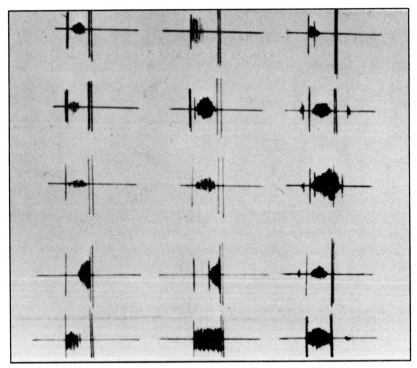

Figure 95: Sketch of various heart sounds and murmurs.

- **Grading Systolic Murmurs** — Grading of systolic murmurs is important and very helpful. They are graded from 1 to 6 based on a system introduced by the late Samuel A. Levine:

Grade 1 is the faintest murmur that one hears with the stethoscope, but often is not detected immediately. Only after the ear is "tuned in" by adjustment of the tips of the stethoscope in the ear or after a few moments of concentration, will a faint systolic murmur be heard.

Grade 2 is also a faint murmur, but one will hear it immediately on placing the stethoscope over the chest.

Grade 3 is still on the faint side, but is louder than the Grade 2 murmur.

On the opposite end of the grading scale, Grade 6 is the loudest murmur and can even be heard with the stethoscope not actually touching the chest wall. Sometimes this murmur can even be heard a few feet from the chest. However, as long as one can see daylight between the stethoscope and the chest wall and still hear a murmur, it is a Grade 6 murmur.

Grade 5 is also a loud murmur, but it is not heard unless the stethoscope is actually touching the chest wall.

Grade 4 is a loud murmur and is a significant jump in intensity from Grade 3. Grade 4 murmurs and above can be accompanied by a palpable systolic thrill.

This grading system is a cardiac pearl that has stood the test of time and is used throughout the world.

- **Intensity of Murmur** — If a palpable systolic thrill is felt, the murmur is at least a Grade 4 intensity (Figure 96).

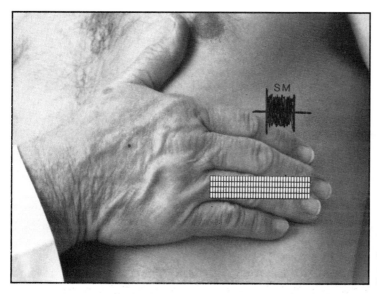

Figure 96: Thrill — The detection of a palpable systolic thrill indicates the presence of a systolic murmur (SM) grade 4 or above.

- **Listen to Areas Other than the Precordium** — We should not limit our auscultation to the heart, but in every patient examined we should listen over the neck, back and anterior chest, abdomen and groin. One can listen over these areas quickly and efficiently. Make it a routine of the physical examination, and it will be rewarding.

(Figure 97) A short systolic murmur heard over multiple areas of the back of the chest and often over the right and left anterior chest may afford the first clue as to the diagnosis of pulmonary branch arterial stenosis.

With very large shunts (3:1 or greater) of atrial septal defect, a systolic murmur similar to the pulmonary arterial branch stenosis may be found over the back, if searched for. An arteriovenous fistula might be detected by the presence of a continuous murmur.

A systolic murmur of coarctation may be heard of almost equal intensity in the upper back as well as the front. Larger intercostal arteries of coarctation and Tetralogy of Fallot may at times be felt and have a systolic murmur. (In Tetralogy patients, a continuous murmur may also be detected over the intercostal arteries.)

The transmitted holosystolic murmur of severe mitral regurgitation can be detected at the left posterior lung base. (The murmur has radiated — "band-like" — from the lower left sternal border, apex, and axillary lines to the posterior lung base.)

Some very musical systolic murmurs are heard at the apex.

- **Cardiac Pearl:** Always rule out aortic stenosis in a patient with the following findings: A very high-pitched musical systolic murmur that peaks in mid-systole and can be heard over the precordium (although it may be detected only at the apex); heart sounds that may be distant or absent (Figure 93).

The patient is usually elderly, male and has an emphysematous chest having an increase in anteroposterior (AP) diameter. With such a murmur, the patient is more likely to have aortic stenosis of milder degrees rather than the severe type, and often not causing symptoms. This same patient can have a more typical harsh murmur of the aortic valve over the carotids in the neck.

Various descriptive terms have been used for this type of systolic murmur, such as "seagull" and "cooing dove". It really is not typical of either bird's cry or call; some use these descriptions for a type of diastolic murmur. It is probably best to discard these terms.

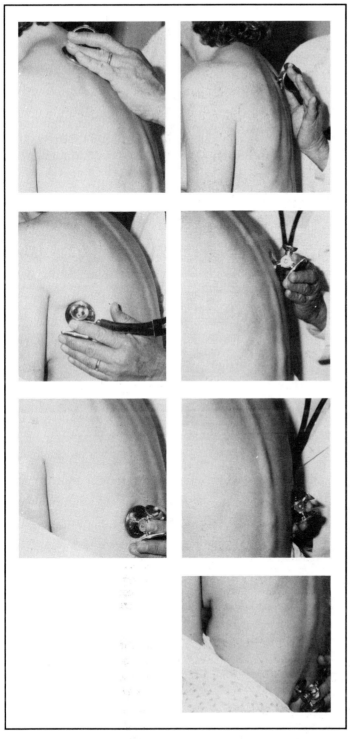

Figure 97: Listening over the back.

- **If one hears a *holosystolic* (or *pansystolic)* murmur that occupies all of systole, think of three conditions: mitral regurgitation, tricuspid regurgitation, and ventricular septal defect. The innocent systolic murmur is not holosystolic.**

Whereas ventricular septal defect is the most common of these three in infants and children, it is the least common in adults and older age. The reason for this is the large number of spontaneous closures of these ventricular defects in childhood, plus those that are surgically corrected. Instead, mitral regurgitation is now the most frequent lesion of the three in adults.

Therefore, in both mitral regurgitation and ventricular septal defect, there is earlier emptying of the blood from the left ventricle with systole, resulting in earlier closure of the aortic component of the second sound, thereby producing a wider split.

Innocent Systolic Murmur — Athlete: Let's say a patient is seen who enjoys marathon running. He has no complaints, is thin and muscular. An early to mid-systolic murmur is present, with normal splitting of the second heart sound. In addition, an intermittent third heart sound was detected. Should this patient continue to participate in long distance running? If these are the only findings, yes.

- **An early to mid-systolic murmur, with normal splitting of the second heart sound, plus an intermittent third heart sound is a perfectly normal finding if there are no other symptoms or signs of heart disease.**

Even though the person may be middle aged, if he is asymptomatic, and has no additional cardiovascular findings on a total evaluation, including electrocardiogram and chest x-ray, the findings are completely within the normal range. There is no need for him to give up the sport he likes.

Some innocent murmurs have a vibratory, somewhat musical buzzing quality. They may sound like a tuning fork that is set in vibration. This vibratory type of innocent murmur is called Still's murmur, named after George Frederick Still (Common Disorders and Diseases of Childhood, London: Frode, Hodder and Stroughton, 1909).

- **When, in a young person, you hear a grade 1 to 3 vibratory, somewhat musical systolic murmur occupying the first to middle part of systole, you should be immediately reassured that this is probably an innocent murmur of Still's type.**

The following is excerpted from Dr. Still's description of the murmur that bears his name:

"And here I should like to draw attention to a particular bruit which has somewhat of a musical character, but neither of sinister omen nor does it indicate endocarditis of any sort. In my own notebooks I am in the habit of labeling it physiologic bruit, but only for want of some better name. It is heard usually just below the level of the nipple and about halfway between the left margin of the sternum and the vertical nipple line; it is not heard in the axilla nor behind; it is systolic and is often so small that only a careful observer would detect it; moreover, it is sometimes very variable in audibility, being scarcely noticeable with some beats and easily heard with others; its characteristic feature is a twanging sound, very like that made by twanging a piece of tense string. This bruit is found mostly in children between the ages of 2 and 6 years; as a rule... the bruit is discovered only in the course of routine examination. It persists sometimes for many months. Have noted it as present in one case for two years. Whatever may be its origin, I think it is... not due to any organic disease of the heart, either congenital or acquired; and I mention it in connection with endocarditis because I have seen several cases in which it has given rise not only to groundless alarm, but to unnecessary restriction, so that the child has been treated as an invalid and not allowed to walk about."

Dr. Still's observations are of historical interest and value. His advice concerning "unnecessary restriction" still applies, eight decades later. One wishes it were possible to ask Dr. Still if any of the musical vibratory murmurs were in late systole, particularly those that were "sometimes very variable in audibility, being scarcely noticeable with some beats and easily heard with others." Of course today this would suggest mitral valve prolapse in which variability of the "systolic whoop" or "honk" is common (Figure 98). Almost certainly this is what Dr. Still was referring to, since an innocent murmur, while it can become louder with exercise, excitement, or fever, does not vary from beat to beat. Such variability is sometimes characteristic of mitral valve prolapse.

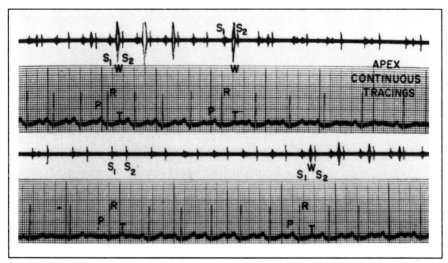

Figure 98: Mitral Valve Prolapse — Note inconstant late musical murmur (whoop-W) which comes and goes. The midsystolic click does the same.

Diastolic Murmurs

- **Aortic diastolic murmurs can be loud and be caused by varying etiologies. They can be associated with a palpable thrill along the third left sternal border. Sometimes the murmur has a "to and fro" quality, loud with a very low, somewhat musical quality. On the other hand, the murmur may be very loud with very predominant high frequency components (Figure 99). Sometimes the diastolic murmur resembles sawing wood, with the loud component being in diastole.**

- **Intermittent Murmurs: Aortic diastolic murmurs from aortic regurgitation, sometimes with musical components, may be heard intermittently.**

  This is uncommon but has been described in patients with luetic (syphilitic) aortic insufficiency. It is postulated that an aortic cusp occasionally becomes everted and causes the transient intermittent aortic regurgitation. Intermittent murmurs have also occurred with prosthetic valves that have a moving part. For example, a disc may get temporarily stuck, thereby producing a systolic (or less likely a diastolic) murmur. The term "cocked" disc has been used to describe this.

- **Pregnancy — A faint grade 1 or 2 early, blowing diastolic murmur of aortic regurgitation might not be detected in a pregnant woman, particularly in her last trimester.**

  If a woman has not been examined before her pregnancy, this diastolic murmur might not be detected; it should be carefully searched for after completion of her pregnancy.

- **Remember, also, that almost all pregnant ladies have an innocent grade 2 or 3, early to mid systolic murmur, which may not be heard before or after her pregnancy (Figures 100 and 101).**

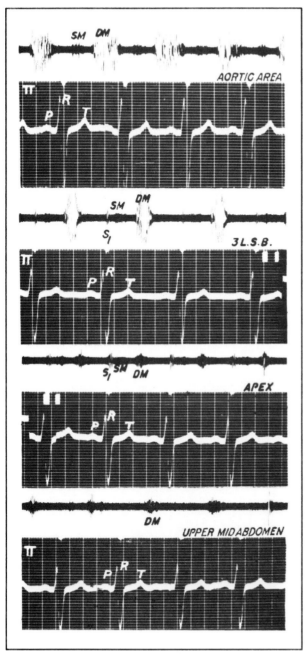

Figure 99: Luetic Heart Disease — A loud musical diastolic murmur (DM) is best heard over the aortic and third left sternal border. A systolic murmur (SM) is also detected. Note the diastolic murmur is loud enough to be heard over the mid abdomen.

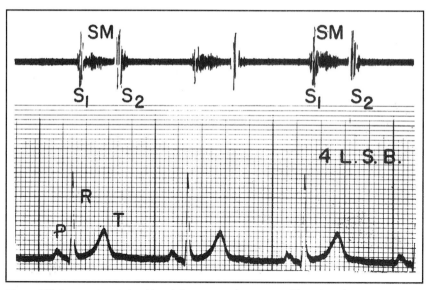

Figure 100: Innocent early to mid-systolic murmur of pregnancy. There is no heart disease present.

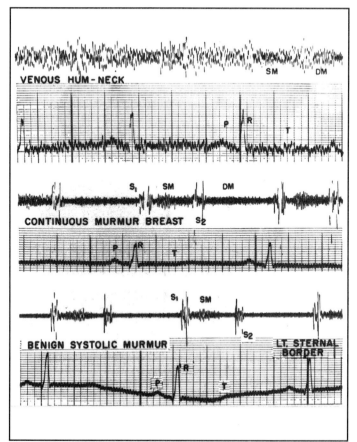

Figure 101: Some Auscultatory Findings of Pregnancy — Most pregnant women have innocent venous hums in the neck and innocent systolic murmurs. Sometimes a continuous innocent murmur can occur over an engorged non-nursing breast, though it is more likely in a nursing one.

An innocent venous hum over the neck is also an expected finding, particularly in the last trimester. Uncommonly, a continuous murmur can be heard over an engorged breast(s) of pregnancy — usually a nursing breast, but not always. It can be often eliminated by pressure with a finger over the area; if this mammary hum is over the left breast, it can be misinterpreted as patent ductus or as an arteriovenous fistula over either breast. Of course, it disappears after pregnancy or cessation of nursing.

- **Minimal Murmur of Aortic Insufficiency — Good Life Expectancy. It is very probable that a patient having only a minimal aortic regurgitation, manifested by a faint grade 1 or 2 aortic diastolic murmur, can be completely asymptomatic as far as the heart is concerned; if that amount of leak persists unchanged, the patient could lead a normal physically active life, and with a normal life span. However if a greater degree of leak develops, symptoms and signs of left ventricular enlargement occur.**

    This type of murmur may be heard with a bicuspid aortic valve (Figure 102). It is known that some of the valves never worsen throughout life; others are more likely to show progression with the passage of time.

- **The faint grade 1 or 2 aortic diastolic murmur of a congenital bicuspid aortic valve is frequently overlooked. Infective endocarditis following simple dental extractions, cleaning, or filling may affect the valve, damage it and produce wide-open severe aortic regurgitation requiring valve replacement at surgery.**

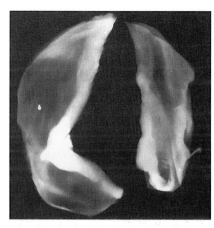

Figure 102: A Congenital Bicuspid Aortic Valve — Note one cusp is larger. This valve caused pure aortic regurgitation.

- **The patient with minimal aortic regurgitation often has a lesion that is frequently overlooked: Congenital bicuspid aortic valve. Listen carefully for an early systolic sound which may be the *ejection sound,* a hallmark of such a valve (Figure 103). Such a patient will almost certainly have an aortic ejection sound heard at the apex, as well as at the base.**

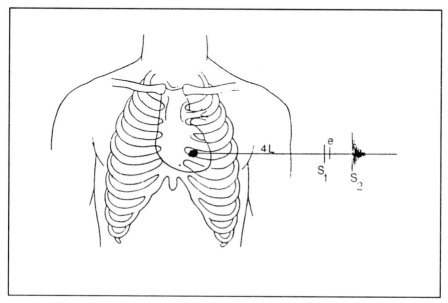

Figure 103: Minimal Regurgitation — A patient with a congenital bicuspid aortic valve having minimal aortic regurgitation. Note faint murmur tailing off of the second sound (S_2). The aortic ejection sound (e) was heard from the apex to the aortic area.

This faint aortic diastolic murmur would almost certainly not be overlooked if the physician listens when the patient is sitting upright, leaning forward, breath held in deep expiration; firm pressure should be exerted on the diaphragm of the stethoscope against the chest wall to produce an imprint of the stethoscope on the skin, as already discussed.

If the patient's faint murmur is diagnosed, then appropriate antibiotic prophylaxis, as suggested by the American Heart Association, should be given (See page 83).

- **Antibiotic prophylaxis should be given to patients with valvular heart disease. The most common causes of infective endocarditis are dental procedures and heart valve replacement. Antibiotic prophylaxis is indi-**

cated not only for extractions of teeth, but also for simpler procedures such as cleaning and filling. Infective endocarditis has been definitely documented to occur with these simpler procedures.

Occasionally one hears a very high-pitched, somewhat musical, faint diastolic murmur that is prolonged and persists through one-half to two thirds of diastole. In my experience, these are most likely to occur in the patient who has systolic hypertension and minimal aortic leak. The diastolic blood pressure is not reduced, or only slightly so. Perhaps it is the pressure head of an increased diastolic blood pressure that causes this prolongation of the faint murmur.

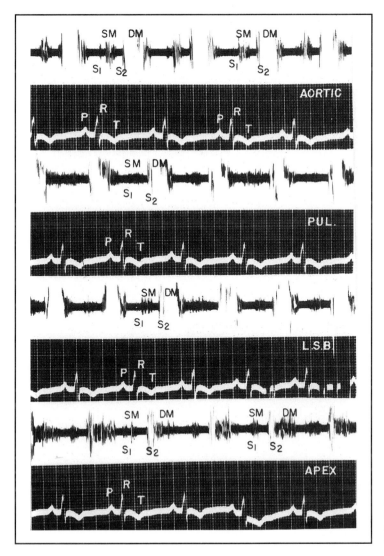

Figure 104: "Cooing Dove" Murmur: Note loud, musical, diastolic murmur heard over precordium from aortic to apical areas, caused by severe luetic aortic insufficiency.

- **Horses may have musical aortic diastolic murmurs, and some are apparently related to congenital bands that are present below the aortic valve, which vibrate in the presence of a leaking aortic valve.**

A "cooing dove" murmur has been described by some as being a musical systolic murmur, whereas others have described it as being a diastolic murmur. Figure 104 shows a patient with such a *diastolic* murmur.

- **Mitral Stenosis With a Diastolic "Whine"** — Occasionally, a patient who has a tight mitral stenosis will have the following findings: A loud first sound, a high frequency "whine" tailing off the second sound and ending about mid-diastole, an opening snap, and a diastolic rumble occupying all of diastole, with a presystolic accentuation (Figure 104A).

The etiology of this unusual murmur may be a minimal aortic regurgitation. The fact that it may be heard at the apex mitigates against the etiology being pulmonary valve regurgitation.

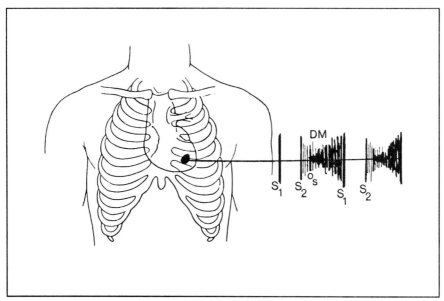

Figure 104A: Whine Murmur – Patient with a "tight" mitral stenosis having a diastolic rumble following the opening snap that occupies all of diastole and with presystolic accentuation. In addition, an early aortic diastolic "whine" murmur is heard.

Mitral Valve Prolapse

Mitral valve prolapse is synonymous with other terms such as:
Systolic click-murmur syndrome
Billowing mitral valve leaflet syndrome
Floppy valve syndrome
Barlow's syndrome
The basic pathology is so-called myxomatous degeneration of the mitral valve. The mitral valve is made up of two basic components: a fibrosa element and a spongiosa element. In this condition the spongiosa element proliferates. Excessive leaflet tissue can cause a scalloping or hooding effect of the valve. There may be thinning and elongation of the chordae tendineae as shown in Figure 105. Tricuspid valve prolapse also occurs (Figure 106).

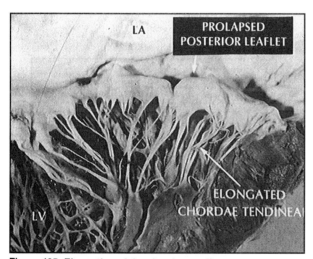

Figure 105: Elongation of the chordae tendineae.

- **Detecting Mitral Valve Prolapse — Mitral valve prolapse often is first diagnosed by echocardiogram. Your stethoscope, however, is still the best instrument to detect and diagnose prolapse of the mitral valve.**

Both the echocardiogram and angiogram can fail to document prolapse. It also can be missed by the stethoscope; however, generally that is because the physician is

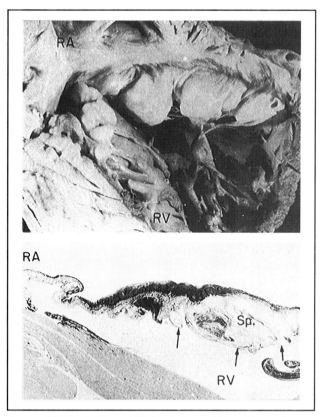

Figure 106 A/B: A. Tricuspid Valve Prolapse. Tricuspid valve in a 79-year-old woman with a floppy mitral valve, pulmonary emphysema and cor pulmonale. Each leaflet is thickened, opaque and prolapsed into the right atrium (RA): RV = right ventricle.

B. Photomicrograph of the tricuspid valve in a 65-year-old man with a floppy mitral valve. RA = right atrial cavity; RV = right ventricular cavity. The spongiosa (SP) of the peripheral part of the leaflet is increased and invades and disrupts the fibrosa (arrows). There is an extensive fibroelastic deposit on the right atrial surface of the leaflet and localized fibrous deposits on the right ventricular surface of the leaflet. A right ventricular friction lesion covers the myocardium near the base of the valve. (Elastic tissue stain, X5)

not "mentally set" to listen specifically for the typical auscultatory findings, or has not listened carefully in a quiet room with the patient in the following positions:

    Supine
    Turned to the left lateral position
    Sitting
    Standing
    Squatting
    Also, you may need to employ other bedside maneuvers — such as the Valsalva
    As a rule, findings of mitral valve prolapse on auscultation are best detected using the flat diaphragm chest piece of the stethoscope. The auscultatory findings of

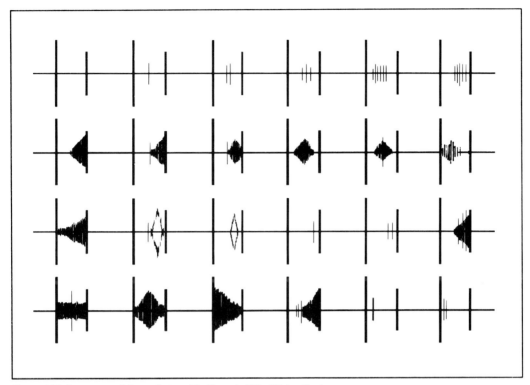

Figure 107: Spectrum of Auscultatory Findings in Mitral Valve Prolapse.

this condition represent a fascinating spectrum (Figures 107 and 108). We must listen very carefully to our patients since, in some, the telltale auscultatory findings are heard only on inspiration, in others only on expiration. The findings may be transient, intermittent, varying at times, with some heartbeats having:

No click or murmur
Only a click or clicks
Only a murmur
Combinations of click and murmur
A musical murmur termed "whoop" or "honk"

The great majority of patients with mitral valve prolapse are completely asymptomatic and need no treatment. Reassurance as to their good prognosis may be all that is required. Some patients have palpitations and a degree of chest discomfort. Occasionally sedatives, beta blockers and antiarrhythmics are needed and may be effective in treatment, although some patients are not helped by these drugs.

The most serious complication is rupture of a chorda tendinea, which may occur spontaneously or as a result of infective endocarditis on the valve. Endocarditis can damage the valve, resulting in acute mitral regurgitation. Surgery may be necessary for correction of the significant mitral regurgitation resulting from these complications; however, this represents a small minority of the large number of patients who have mitral valve prolapse.

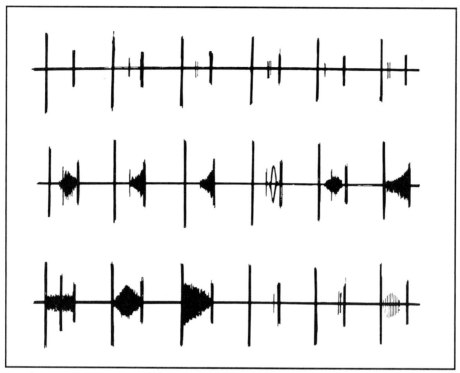

Figure 108: Mitral Valve Prolapse — More examples of the range of possible auscultatory findings in patients with mitral valve prolapse. Findings may even vary from time to time in the same patient.

● Complications and Associated Findings of Mitral Valve Prolapse:

1. Progressive, increasingly severe mitral regurgitation.
2. Ruptured chordae tendineae (infective endocarditis, idiopathic).
3. Rupture of valve leaflet (trauma, infective endocarditis, idiopathic).
4. Calcification of mitral annulus.
5. Transient ischemic attacks. Cerebral emboli.
6. Arrhythmias.
7. Chest pain.
8. In some patients, symptoms compatible with neurocirculatory asthenia (Da Costa's syndrome, effort syndrome).
9. Anxiety.
10. Cardiac neurosis.
11. Sudden death (rare).

Prognosis is excellent for most patients with mitral valve prolapse. This should be stressed to our patients because many know about their condition and have unnecessary fears and anxieties concerning it. Unfortunately, a number have been told about very rare complications such as sudden death; we know that this has occurred, but it is rare and has been overemphasized.

- **Prophylaxis Against Infective Endocarditis** — Patients with mitral valve prolapse may develop infective endocarditis with resultant severe mitral regurgitation. Antibiotic prophylaxis, as outlined by the American Heart Association (see page 83), is therefore recommended to our patients having dental procedures, various surgical procedures, and some diagnostic procedures of the gastrointestinal and urogenital tracts.

Some years ago we had five patients (not with mitral valve prolapse) within a period of 22 months who had proven infective endocarditis due to Streptococcus viridans following cleaning and/or filling of teeth (no extractions). Three of them died of the complications of the endocarditis. Therefore, as we said previously, we recommend antibiotic prophylaxis for all dental procedures, including cleaning, filling and extraction, in patients with mitral valve prolapse.

- **Sudden death due to mitral valve prolapse is rare.**

It does occur, of course, but in the past this dire event has been overemphasized, and some articles written for lay consumption have focused unnecessarily on it. This has caused undue anxiety in the many patients in our country who have this common condition (perhaps 15 million).

Imagine an irresponsible medical reporter who attended a medical conference and then wrote a column in his newspaper with the headline, "Heart Condition Causes Death." This was the sensational bit of information about this condition that he gleaned from his attendance at the conference. Also imagine the harm that was done to the patients with the condition who read this account. Undue fears and anxieties were bound to occur in many who knew they had this condition.

The outlook is excellent in the great majority of patients. Most are essentially asymptomatic and 90% of patients who have mitral valve prolapse require only information and reassurance. It is better to stress the true, positive aspects of this condition; the rare possibility of sudden death should not be emphasized.

- **Palpitations** — If one has a patient in their 20s or 30s who complains of palpitation that could be due to frequent premature beats or episodes of paroxysmal atrial tachycardia or paroxysmal atrial fibrillation, be sure to consider the possibility of mitral valve prolapse.

This appears to be more common in women than men (although, of course, it does occur in men). Also, some women with mitral valve prolapse have such palpitations only when they are pregnant. Though mitral valve prolapse can occur in children, teenagers and older patients, consider the possibility of mitral valve prolapse especially in the young adults just described.

Figures 109 A, B, C, D, E show the various arrhythmias that can occur with mitral valve prolapse. The most frequent are benign premature ventricular contractions. Many patients are unaware or are not bothered by them. No treatment (except reassurance) is usually necessary.

- **Seldom Recognized Variant of Mitral Valve Prolapse — Systolic clicks generally occur in mid to late systole. However, a seldom recognized variant of mitral valve prolapse is that they can occur in early to mid systole; they can be multiple and rapid and can simulate the flipping of a deck of cards or the creaking of new leather. Once one has heard this variant of mitral valve prolapse, it should be accurately diagnosed in others.** (Figures 107, 108)

This variant is also different in that these clicks are usually better heard over the third left sternal border and pulmonic area rather than the lower left sternal border and apex. Although I have seen about 100 patients having this variant (also documented on echocardiography) I have not seen it reported in the medical literature.

It can simulate and be misdiagnosed as a pericardial friction rub because of these multiple rapid sounds in systole. However, if we remember the cardiac pearl of friction rubs, this confusion should not occur:

- **A pericardial friction rub has 2 or 3 components rather than only one in systole: (1) the atrial systolic, (2) the ventricular systolic, and (3) the ventricular diastolic.**

- **Systolic "Whoop" — A very loud, musical systolic murmur — a "whoop" — occurring in the last half of systole is most likely due to mitral valve prolapse (Figure 110).**

Many years ago, a 23-year-old woman from another state was sitting outside of my office. On questioning her, she said, "I've come for the operation." I had no correspondence concerning her, but on examining her, she had no symptoms referable to her heart or cardiovascular system. On physical examination, the only positive finding was an intermittent, loud musical murmur occurring in the latter part of systole. It reminded me of the sound that occurs with a child who has whooping cough.

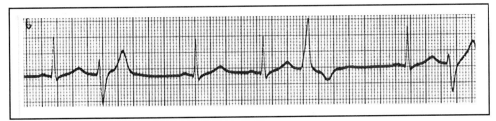

Figure 109A: Premature ventricular contractions.

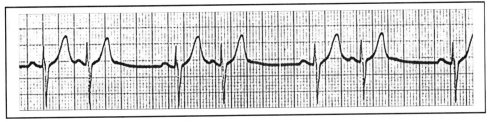

Figure 109B: Premature atrial contractions.

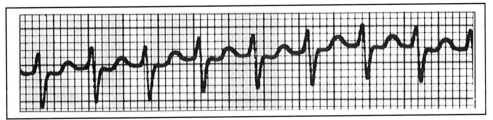

Figure 109C: Paroxysmal atrial tachycardia.

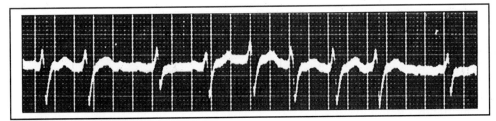

Figure 109D: Atrial fibrillation.

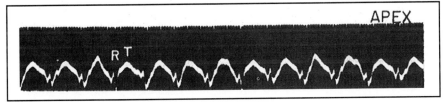

Figure 109E: Ventricular tachycardia.

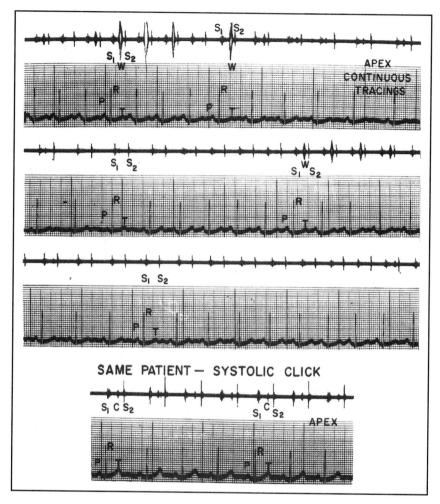

Figure 110: Systolic Whoop — Note intermittent musical systolic whoop (W). At times, systole is clear of sounds or clicks (panel third from top). At other times only a click (C) is heard.

Thus, we gave it the name "systolic whoop" and believed it was a benign finding, even though at that time we could not explain its origin. Sometimes she would have no whoop sound, but would have a midsystolic click or clicks, and at still other times she had a late apical systolic murmur that did not have the musical "whoop" character. Subsequently, with the passage of years, this was documented as being a part of the spectrum of auscultatory findings of mitral valve prolapse. Obviously no surgery was required.

Once this peculiar new sound had been described, others recognized and identified it in their own patients. Since then, we have seen many patients who have these musical "whoop" murmurs.

Subsequently, physicians at Duke University described a sound of similar nature and they termed it "systolic honk." Obviously more goose hunting is done in

132

North Carolina than in the Washington, D.C. area. A "systolic whoop" can also be caused by a prolapse of the tricuspid valve. However, today the term "whoop" may not be a truly descriptive term, since most medical students have never seen and heard a patient with whooping cough and therefore would not know what the whoop of that disease is like. Neither, I suspect, have most heard the "honk" of a goose.

Sometimes a late musical systolic "whoop" or "honk" may be a constant finding, or, more commonly, intermittently heard. Only very recently I saw a patient with mitral valve prolapse who had an intermittent "scraping" sound (like a metal blade scraping another metal) in late systole. These are variants of mitral valve prolapse and might only be heard in different positions.

The systolic "whoop" can be very loud; in fact, loud enough that others can hear it even several feet away. Several anecdotes: A woman "panicked" when she first heard loud noises emitting from her husband's chest (while in bed).

A young lady who was kind enough to be a patient we presented in some of our teaching conferences (group auscultation) would amuse the physicians in attendance by stating that the intermittent chest noise of her tricuspid valve might give a boyfriend the wrong impression that she cared for him more than she really did.

Another patient had such a loud late systolic whoop that she stopped coming to the cardiac clinic because of her embarrassing chest noise, which occurred with exertion; on climbing the stairs and boarding the subway people were aghast. However, she remarked, "I always got a seat."

Only recently, several residents told me about a peculiar sound that they were hearing in a patient; they had never heard anything like it before. The patient had an intermittent faint, but definite, "squeak" (like a mouse), in the latter part of systole. This was one of the many variants of mitral valve prolapse. Once hearing it, it will be readily identified when hearing it in another patient.

- **Differentiating Mitral Valve Prolapse from Innocent Systolic Murmur — This differentiation generally is not difficult. The typical murmur of mitral valve prolapse is in mid to late systole, whereas the innocent murmur is in the early to mid portions of systole. A click (or clicks) frequently accompanies the murmur of mitral valve prolapse but is absent with an innocent murmur.**

There are exceptions, of course. Occasionally, murmurs of mitral valve prolapse are heard in early or mid-systole with or without an associated click or clicks. The *squatting maneuver* is valuable in bringing out these systolic clicks and murmurs (generally late apical), because they can be altered on squatting.

At times, the squatting maneuver can also cause movement of clicks and/or murmurs in systole as a result of this change in position. A maneuver that increases volume to the left side of the heart, such as squatting, may delay these auscultatory findings, and therefore the click or murmur may move closer to the second heart sound (Figure 111). On prompt standing and with a decrease in volume they may move in the opposite direction in systole — closer to the first heart sound. Also contributing is the bending of the knees and hips, which can increase peripheral arterial systolic pressure, and cause movement closer to the second sound, and closer to the first sound on standing.

The fact that there is a *change* of these auscultatory findings serves as additional evidence of the diagnosis of mitral valve prolapse. In some patients the clicks and/or murmur might not be heard in either the standing or squatting positions.

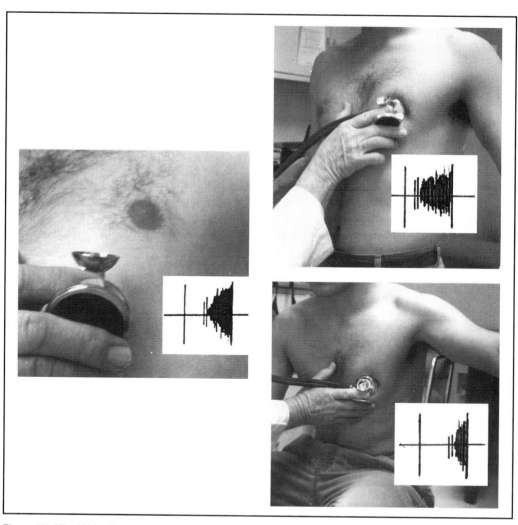

Figure 111: Mitral Valve Prolapse — Movement of clicks and murmurs with change of position.
Left: Patient lying on back. Note two systolic clicks in mid systole followed by late apical systolic murmur (SM). On standing (top right), the clicks move toward the first sound (S₁) as does the murmur, which becomes longer and often louder. On squatting (bottom right) the clicks and murmur move toward the second sound.

- **Complications** — The most serious and frequent complication of mitral valve prolapse is rupture of a chorda tendinea. This may occur spontaneously or with infective endocarditis (probably 50% chance of either).

Mitral valve prolapse is a very common occurrence. Probably 90% of patients are completely asymptomatic and therefore often unaware that they have this condition. Their outlook for a normal life is excellent.

Any of the wide variety of auscultatory events may, with rupture of chordae tendinea, produce a holosystolic murmur peaking in midsystole and decreasing in the latter part of systole (see Figure 112). For example, a patient may have only one or more systolic clicks and have no symptom whatsoever; with rupture of a chorda tendinea the patient will develop a significant leak of his or her mitral valve, which then produces varying degrees of mitral regurgitation, including acute pulmonary edema. In many, this may necessitate mitral valve surgery and/or replacement.

- **Ejection Sound Terminology** — It is suggested that the term "systolic click" be reserved for and identified with mitral valve prolapse. In other circumstances, rather than the term "systolic ejection click", use ejection *sound*. This terminology is clearer and more precise.

- It has been my policy to give antibiotic prophylaxis to all patients with mitral valve prolapse — including those having a click, or clicks (no murmur), as well as those patients with a systolic murmur.

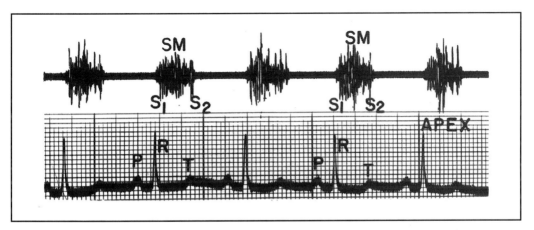

Figure 112: Rupture: Typical systolic murmur (SM) of rupture of a major chorda tendinea. Note decrease in murmur in the latter part of systole.

Some authorities recommend prophylaxis only for the patient who has a systolic murmur with the prolapse, stating that it is not indicated with those who have only a click or clicks. However, I disagree with this, because I can cite many patients with mitral valve prolapse that have transient systolic murmurs as well as clicks. Also, I have personally observed patients who have had documented infective endocarditis where only a single click or several clicks had been present, and who never had a systolic murmur of the prolapse. It is also well known that one can examine a patient with mitral valve prolapse on one occasion and hear only a click or clicks; on another examination, the typical late apical systolic murmur (which may or may not be associated with clicks) is also present. At still other times in the same patient, no murmur or clicks are heard.

Also, on continuous recordings of the phonocardiogram, we have verified findings varying from no murmur or click to clicks, murmurs, whoops, honks, etc., which may be transient and intermittent.

- **Overdiagnosis and Underdiagnosis by Echocardiography — Some patients are diagnosed as having mitral valve prolapse because of misinterpretation of the echocardiogram.**

We have seen a fair number of such patients. If a careful search for auscultatory findings of mitral valve prolapse fails to find any, repeat echocardiograms may also fail to show mitral valve prolapse.

A recent example was a 16-year-old high school football player who was evaluated because of a question as to whether he should play. History revealed that the echocardiogram taken by his physician was quoted as showing mitral valve prolapse. On physical examination, the patient was entirely asymptomatic and all findings were normal. When listening for auscultatory findings consistent with mitral valve prolapse, none were found. The echocardiogram was repeated at our institution with instructions to take extra time to search for any possibility of prolapse; the echocardiogram was completely normal. This made the decision about playing football quite easy.

The echocardiogram has been very useful in detecting mitral valve prolapse, but even in the best of hands, the echocardiogram may miss (or as pointed out previously, overdiagnose) mitral valve prolapse. When we were both participating in a medical symposium, I asked one of the country's experts in echocardiography how often echocardiography might miss the detection of mitral valve prolapse. He answered, "In about ten percent." I have seen many patients with mitral valve prolapse detected by the stethoscope, in whom the echocardiography was interpreted as being normal. I have also seen a number of patients whose echocardiogram had initially been reported as negative, but the clinical auscultatory findings were diagnostic of prolapse, and on repeat echocardiogram positive findings of this condition were found.

- **Misuse of Echocardiography** — Echocardiography is often unnecessary or used for the wrong purpose.

Personally observed have been requests for a color Doppler echocardiogram and on the request sheet under "Reason for Request" was written "question murmur." I have been told of similar situations in other echocardiographic laboratories.

One's stethoscope is the obvious and accurate answer to determining the cause of most murmurs. The aforementioned Reason for Request emphasizes the great need in medicine today to emphasize the basics of cardiovascular evaluation, the Five Finger approach, which includes a careful detailed history and physical examination, electrocardiogram, x-ray and simple laboratory tests that can be done in the physician's office or at the bedside. We need to bring the *patient* from the "back burner" up to the front.

- **Once the diagnosis of mitral valve prolapse is established and the patient remains asymptomatic, frequent repeat echocardiograms are generally not indicated. This only adds undue expense and should be discouraged.**

- **Positions for Auscultation — To detect or rule out mitral valve prolapse, listen to the patient in various positions. Listen with the patient lying flat; turned to the left lateral position and listening over the point of maximum impulse of the left ventricle, the pulmonic area, third left sternal border, lower left sternal border, and apex. Also listen over these same areas with the patient sitting, standing, and squatting.**

- **Cardiac Pearl: Do not exclude mitral valve prolapse until you have listened in all of these positions.**

It is also important to listen in the different phases of respiration. Sometimes clicks and/or murmurs may appear only with inspiration; other times only with expiration. Sometimes they may be heard only in one position, such as the left lateral position, elicited over the apex.

Mitral Valve Prolapse — Chest Anomalies

When we find on examination of our patients that there is a chest anomaly such as straight back (Figures 113 and 114), pectus excavatum (Figure 115), pectus coronatum (Figure 116), or chest asymmetry, we have a clue that mitral valve prolapse might be present. Perhaps 50% of patients with such anomalies may have mitral valve prolapse.

Pectus excavatum was described by Dr. William Evans of London as saucer, cup or funnel types.

● **A patient having the cup or funnel pectus can have the heart in the PA view displaced to the left (Figures 117, 118 and 119), showing little or no cardiac shadow on the right of the spine and a cardiac silhouette that can be misinterpreted as being enlarged. When one sees only this PA chest film, one can suspect pectus even before examining the patient.**

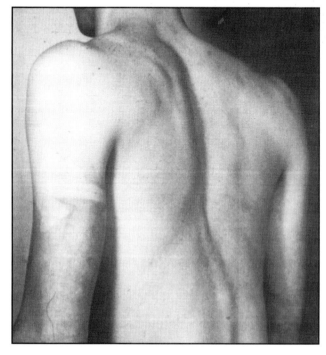

Figure 113: Straight back.

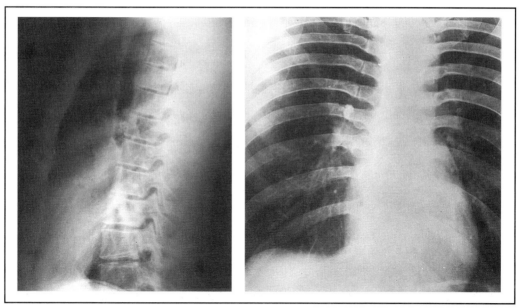

Figure 114: Straight Back — Left: Note "straight back" spine. In fact, it curves anteriorly rather than the usual normal posteriorly. The PA chest film (right) may show a "pancake" shape due to some compression of the heart between the spine and anterior chest wall.

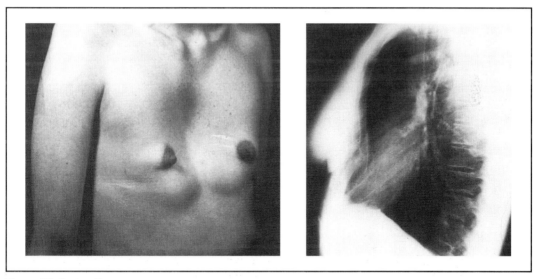

Figure 115: Pectus Excavatum.

● **Cardiac Pearl:** These chest anomalies that cause compression on the heart cause no symptoms. Occasionally surgery for pectus is performed — purely for cosmetic reasons.

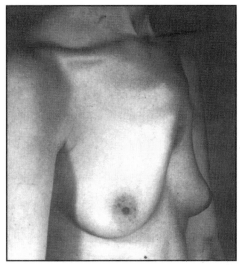

Figure 116: Pectus Coronatum.

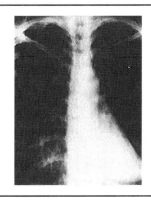

Figure 117: Suspect pectus excavatum when PA view shows little or no cardiac silhouette to right of spine as heart is displaced to left.

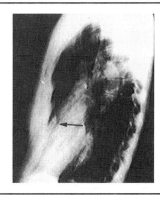

Figure 118: Lateral view shows pectus excavatum.

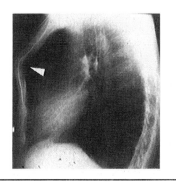

Figure 119: Pectus Coronatum — The patient is a 30-year-old man with a congenital heart disease — pectus coronatum (arrow). He also has a mid-systolic click of mitral valve prolapse.

It is not unusual for me to be asked to evaluate a patient diagnosed as having mitral valve prolapse. A systolic click has been described. On examination, the "click" is in very early systole, which clinically is very unusual; actually it is the second (tricuspid) component of the splitting of the first heart sound that may have "clicking" of a higher frequency than usual. The squatting maneuver (as previously described) is useful; if no movement of this sound occurs, it is unlikely to be mitral valve prolapse.

Hypertrophic Cardiomyopathy

Now let's shake hands again with another patient, and then place our palpating fingers over the radial pulse (Figure 120). We note a quick rise of the pulse; this is called a "flip". It is a sensation obtained when one flips the middle finger of one hand against the middle finger of the other (Figure 121). This brief contact against the stationary finger produces a sensation which we have termed a flip. Even a little flip produces a quick-rise sensation. The quick-rise pulse (also termed Corrigan's or waterhammer pulse) is consistent with aortic regurgitation, a diagnostic possibility to be ruled in or out.

Now, searching for the aortic diastolic murmur, we listen with the patient sitting upright, leaning forward, and breath held in deep expiration. We listen with the flat diaphragm of the stethoscope pressed firmly against the chest wall at the third left sternal border. We expect to hear the early blowing diastolic murmur of aortic regurgitation; however, we don't hear it. Instead there is a *systolic* murmur. Even at this point, we should think of hypertrophic cardiomyopathy (Figure 122). The next step is to use the squatting maneuver. On squatting, the murmur decreases in intensity (on rare occasions it may even disappear) (Figure 123). The murmur becomes louder again on standing, and the diagnosis of hypertrophic cardiomyopathy is made.

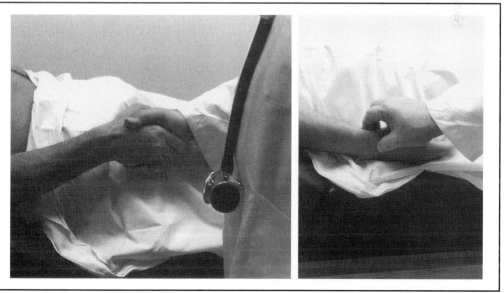

Figure 120: Detecting Hypertrophic Cardiomyopathy — On greeting the patient, shake hands and then palpate the radial pulse.

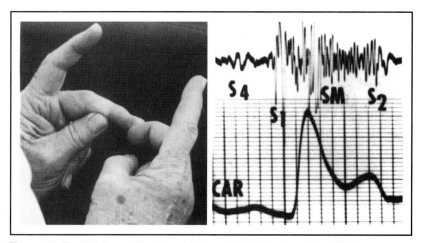

Figure 121: The "flip" sensation of a quick rise arterial pulse of a patient with hypertrophic cardiomyopathy. S_4 = atrial sound; S_1 = first sound; SM = systolic murmur; S_2 = second sound. car = carotid arterial pulse.

This maneuver should be repeated several times, since the characteristic change in the murmur might occur only on the third or fourth time.

- **We term this the "one, two, three, four diagnosis" of hypertrophic cardiomyopathy. Number one: we find a quick rise pulse. Number two: we look for aortic regurgitation. Number 3: we don't find it; instead, a systolic murmur is present. Number four: with the squatting maneuver, the murmur becomes fainter, and on standing again, the murmur gets louder (often even louder than it was originally). This is a superb diagnostic maneuver.**

Most physicians squat as the patient squats, attempting at the same time to listen with the stethoscope. I too used to do this; however, not uncommonly one of us might become unsteady and almost fall into each other (Figure 124). One cannot listen accurately if this awkward situation occurs. After a number of years, it finally dawned on me that there was a simple and more effective way: the physician sits comfortably in a chair (Figure 125). The patient stands facing the physician, steadying himself or herself with the left hand on the examining table. The physician listens with the stethoscope over the patient's left sternal border or apex, thereby obtaining a baseline

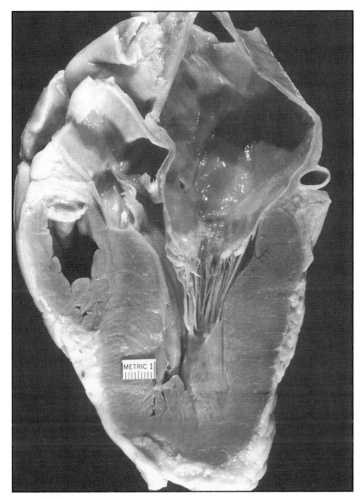

Figure 122: Hypertrophic Cardiomyopathy — Note thickened interventricular septum.

of the auscultatory findings; the patient is then told to squat, and then return to the standing position. This is repeated several times.

Once having used this method of performing the squatting maneuver, I must confess feeling somewhat foolish that I didn't think of it sooner. We term this: The cardiac pearl of the squatting maneuver. The less agile elderly patient can squat and sit on the little stool by the examining table. This works! (This was a suggestion of Dr. James Ronan, one of our faculty members.)

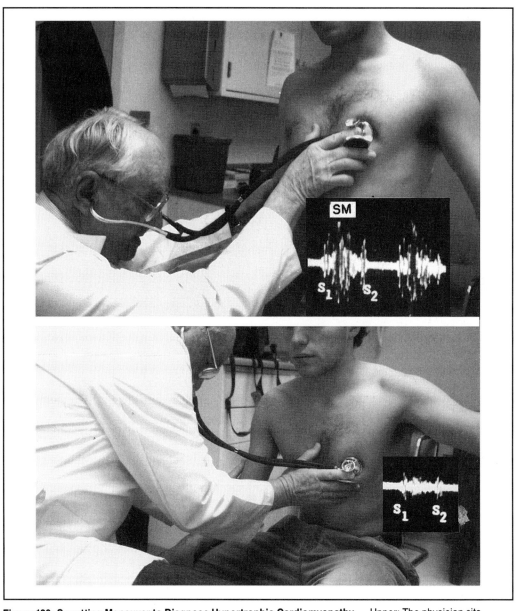

Figure 123: Squatting Maneuver to Diagnose Hypertrophic Cardiomyopathy — Upper: The physician sits comfortably, listening to the patient who at first is standing. The patient, balancing himself with his left hand on the examining table, squats and seats himself on a low stool — a position that bends both his knees and hips. Note systolic murmur (SM) on standing (upper photo) is louder, and on squatting (lower photo) becomes fainter.

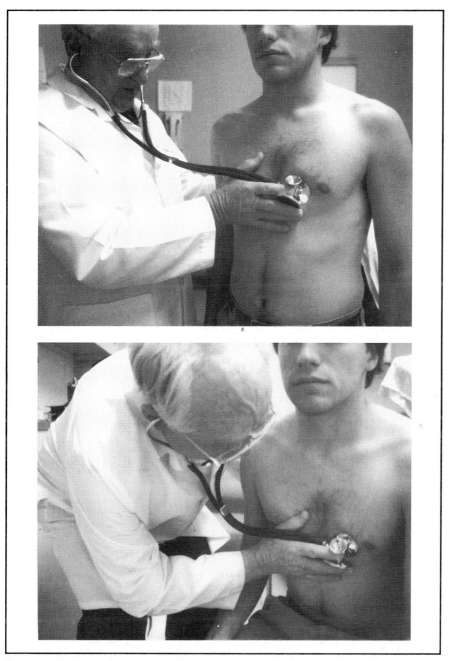

Figure 124: Squatting Maneuver — Wrong Way. The physician stands and squats with the patient. Sometimes unsteadiness results with one or both, causing inadequate concentration on the auscultatory event.

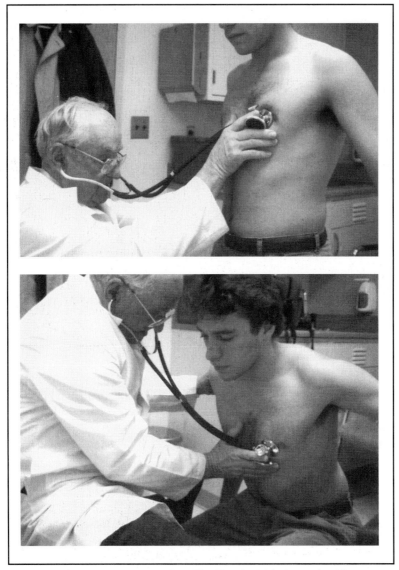

Figure 125: Squatting Maneuver — Best Way. The physician sits comfortably throughout the maneuver. He gets his baseline auscultation with the patient standing. The patient then squats, balancing himself with his left hand on the examining table.

- **The Valsalva maneuver, too, can be helpful in diagnosing hypertrophic cardiomyopathic. While listening along the left sternal border or apex, have the patient take a deep breath, blow the breath out and then strain as if having a bowel movement. The murmur may increase in intensity, indicating a positive response.**

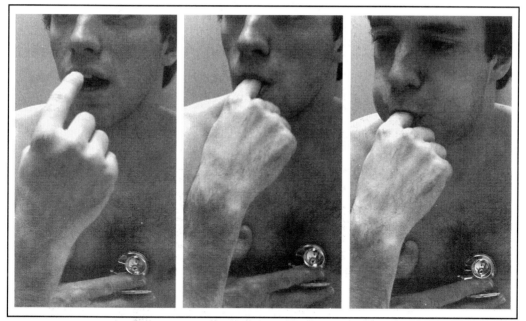

Figure 126: A Simplified, Effective Valsalva Maneuver — The patient places his forefinger in his mouth and seals it with his lips. He is instructed to exhale and, at the point of deep expiration, is told to "blow hard" (right photo). The systolic murmur gets louder.

- **However, some patients, such as the elderly, may have difficulty in performing this maneuver. A simple and efficient way is to have the patient place his index finger in his mouth, seal it with his lips, exhale and at the point of deep expiration, "blow hard" on the finger (Figure 126). This usually works.**

- **Sudden death** in athletes is usually due to ventricular fibrillation.

Under the age of 30, the most likely cause of the fibrillation is hypertrophic cardiomyopathy [formerly termed idiopathic hypertrophic subaortic stenosis (IHSS) or hypertrophic obstructive cardiomyopathy (HOCM)]. Can this condition be "spotted" in a person such as the young athlete? In many the answer is "yes," by looking for it and knowing what we are looking for; and by using the clinical evaluation features including the squatting maneuver as just discussed.

In the international classification of cardiomyopathy, there are three types; hypertrophic cardiomyopathy, dilated cardiomyopathy, and restrictive (or obliterative) cardiomyopathy. The causes are unknown. If the etiology is known, it is a specific cardiomyopathy, such as that related to pregnancy and the post-partum period, alcohol, amyloid, scleroderma, a known virus infection, and others.

- **Precordial Impulse** — With the patient turned to the left lateral position and palpating over the point of maximum impulse of the left ventricle, three impulses may be felt: The presystolic movement and a double systolic impulse. This is called the "triple ripple" impulse associated with hypertrophic cardiomyopathy.

- **Aortic Stenosis vs Hypertrophic Cardiomyopathy** — Although both valvular aortic stenosis and hypertrophic cardiomyopathy can, with more severe degrees of obstruction, produce paradoxical splitting of the second heart sound, it is much more common in patients with hypertrophic cardiomyopathy.

At times, differentiating the systolic murmur of hypertrophic cardiomyopathy from that due to rupture of chordae tendineae can be quite difficult indeed. The ruptured chord murmur may radiate upwards to the base and even be accompanied by a palpable thrill over the base. At times, one hears this murmur, which is originating from the mitral valve, even up into the neck.

- **Cardiac Pearl:** The differentiation of these two similar murmurs: If paradoxical splitting of the second heart sound is present (in the absence of left bundle branch block on the electrocardiogram), the diagnosis should immediately be made of hypertrophic cardiomyopathy.

- **Electrocardiographic Signs of Hypertrophic Cardiomyopathy** — In the absence of any history, symptoms, or signs of coronary artery disease, the presence of significant Q-waves and ST and T-wave changes should alert one to the possibility of hypertrophic cardiomyopathy — particularly in a teenager or young adult.

- A normal electrocardiogram practically rules out the diagnosis of hypertrophic cardiomyopathy. Dilated cardiomyopathy, too, often has some abnormality of the electrocardiogram.

Dilated Cardiomyopathy

- **Etiology — The term "dilated cardiomyopathy" means that the etiology is unknown (Figure 127). However, it is likely that, in the majority of patients with dilated cardiomyopathy, the cause is a virus infection of the heart, even though this was clinically undetected and not proven.**

    Dilated cardiomyopathy has a spectrum of severity varying from mild to severe (Figure 128). It is obvious that if the involvement is mild and diagnosed early, reversion is possible with prompt treatment. On the other hand, if diagnosed late and severe involvement of the myocardium is present, the process may not be improved and death from congestive heart failure and/or ventricular fibrillation results.

- **Although marked restriction of physical activities is a "must", *complete* bed rest is often not necessary in treatment of heart failure associated with myocarditis or dilated cardiomyopathy.**

    It is often unnecessary to have the patient on complete bed rest in the hospital or at home. Instead, what *is* practical is a common sense reduction of physical activities to a significant degree. The patient can be at home, eat meals with the family, watch television, and simply avoid any strenuous physical activity. However, it should be stressed that such restricted activity may be necessary for long periods of time. This is one of the basic ingredients of treatment of acute myocarditis and dilated cardiomyopathy.

    Physical rest can result in reversal of a course that would otherwise almost certainly be progressively downhill.

- **A patient with a mild degree of myocarditis, as can occur with a viral infection, can, following the advice of the practical restriction of physical activities, have reversal to normal.**

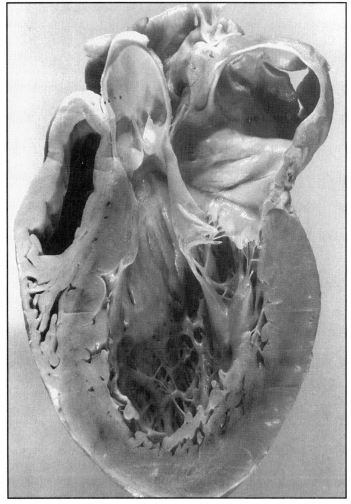

Figure 127: Dilated cardiomyopathy.

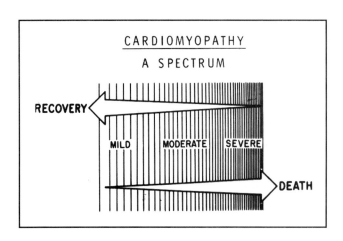

Figure 128: Spectrum of disease in dilated cardiomyopathy. The more severe the involvement the less the chance of regression to normal.

One such patient was employed by the United States Department of State and was stationed overseas in one of the African countries. He developed an acute pericarditis, which was promptly diagnosed and adequately treated. He had a classic clinical history of acute pericarditis. A three component pericardial friction rub (Figure 129) was noted and there were typical S-T wave changes consistent with pericarditis. After approximately five to six weeks, the patient returned to the United States for evaluation and convalescence. Some residual T wave changes on the electrocardiogram were present (Figure 130), but otherwise he was completely asymptomatic. He stated, "I can't wait to get back to my jogging." However, on physical examination, the patient had a subtle pulsus alternans, alternation of the second heart sound, and both atrial (S_4) and ventricular (S_3) diastolic gallops were noted (Figure 131) (See discussion of gallop rhythm relating to heart failure, page 21). These gallop sounds were also very faint but definite. The patient now had signs of mild myocarditis.

The worst thing for this patient would have been to have him resume his daily jogging. Had he done so, it would be likely that at the end of a year a different physician seeing him for the first time might now diagnose dilated cardiomyopathy of moderate to severe degree.

He was a 42-year-old bachelor and lived in a small apartment. His myocarditis was detected very early and his most important treatment was that of restriction of physical activities. Rather than stay in his lonely apartment, alone all day, it was

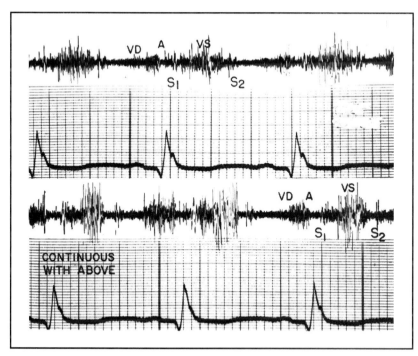

Figure 129: Pericarditis — A patient having a typical 3 component friction rub of acute pericarditis. VS = ventricular systolic component; VD = ventricular diastolic component; A = atrial systolic component. The friction rub is louder in the bottom panel, which is consistent with inspiration.

advised that he come to work each day (which was not of any strenuous physical nature). This would serve to occupy his mind during the day, at night watch television, read, or utilize some such sedentary activities.

This he did and at the end of six weeks he was feeling well. No evidence of myocarditis was present. His pulsus alternans, alternation of sounds and gallop rhythm had completely disappeared. All the changes on the electrocardiogram were normal (Figures 132 and 133). His chest x-ray showed a normal size and silhouette. He is now seven years after the initial examination and I believe he represents a cured acute myocarditis caused by a virus infection.

Had this conservative management *not* been carried out, he could well have progressed to advanced cardiac decompensation and dilated cardiomyopathy.

- **Cardiac Pearl: Patients having acute pericarditis can often have an associated myocarditis. Unless carefully searched for, as in this patient, the myocardial involvement is usually overlooked.**

Subsequently, after a number of months, no evidence of pericarditis is present, but the definite clinical features of advanced, dilated cardiomyopathy are present. A new physician examining the patient at this time might not know of, nor associate the original pericarditis with the present dilated cardiomyopathy, which would now be considered idiopathic (unknown) in etiology.

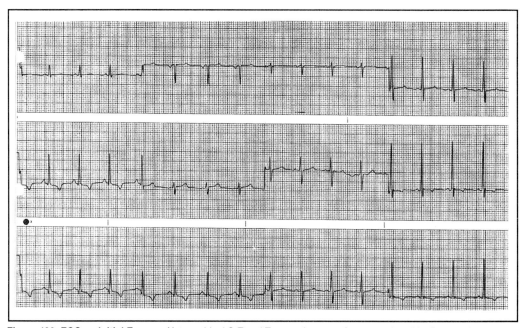

Figure 130: ECG on Initial Exam — Note residual S-T and T wave changes of acute pericarditis. Patient also had subtle but definite findings of myocarditis: pulsus alternans, alternation of intensity of the second sound and a ventricular (S$_3$) diastolic gallop.

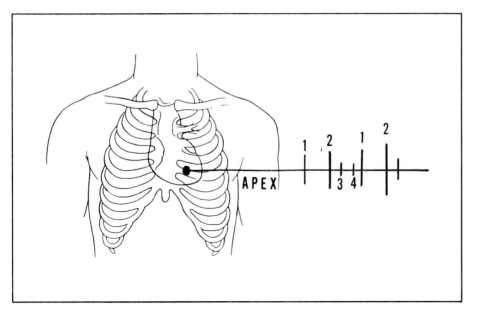

Figure 131: Subtle findings of myocarditis in a patient with resolving pericarditis. Note atrial (S₄) and ventricular (S₃) diastolic gallops. Alternating intensity of heart sounds (1,2) are also present.

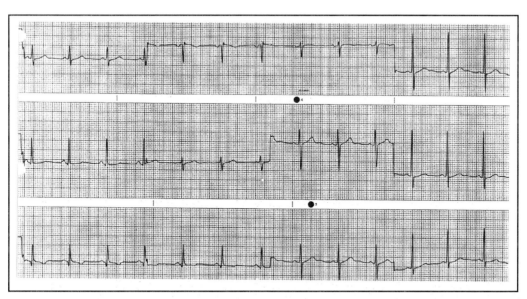

Figure 132: Four Months Later — Note regression of S-T and T wave changes. No pulsus alternans nor alternation of S₂ or ventricular (S₃) gallop are present.

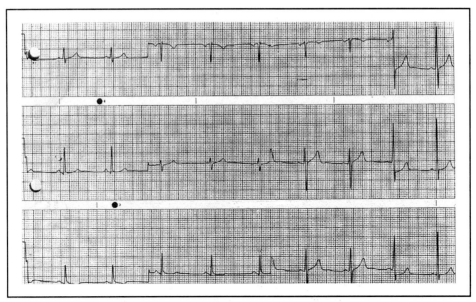

Figure 133: Three Years Later — The ECG continues to be normal (and is so even seven years later), and no evidence of heart disease is present.

Mitral Regurgitation

- **Holosystolic** — A holosystolic (pansystolic) murmur suggests three conditions: mitral regurgitation, tricuspid regurgitation, and ventricular septal defect.

If a murmur is holosystolic, this finding alone immediately takes it out of the ballpark of innocent murmurs, which are early to mid-systolic. If the holosystolic murmur radiates band-like (like a belt) from the lower left sternal border to the apex, anterior mid and posterior axillary lines and even to the posterior lung base, this is diagnostic of mitral regurgitation, usually chronic and of a more advanced degree (Figures 134, 135). If one hears this radiation with the stethoscope, you can almost hang your hat on this diagnosis.

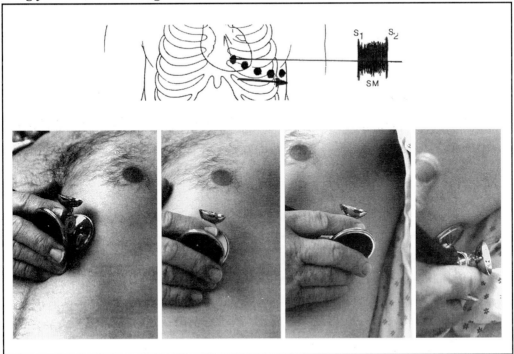

Figure 134: "Band-like" radiation of a holosystolic murmur (SM) from the lower left sternal area (left) to the left axillary areas (right) and posterior lung base is characteristic of mitral regurgitation.

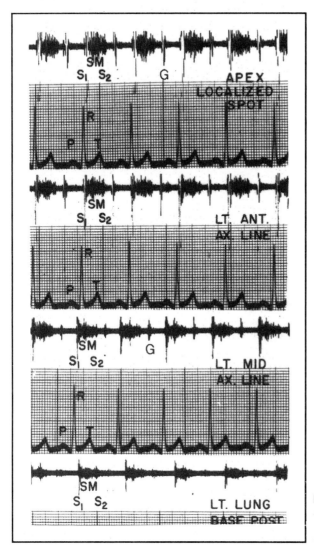

Figure 135: Note "band-like" radiation of holosystolic murmur (SM) from apex to left posterior lung base. Third heart sound gallop (G) was also present.

Some years ago, Drs. Jesse Edwards and Howard Burchell of the Mayo Clinic made observations on the radiation of the murmur of mitral regurgitation relating to whether the pathology involved the anterior or posterior leaflets of the affected valve:

- **Radiation of the Systolic Murmur of Mitral Regurgitation — With significant posterior leaflet damage, the radiation is anterior, upward over the precordium to the base; if anterior leaflet damage predominates, then the radiation is apt to be posterior, from the apex to the axillary lines and posterior lung base.**

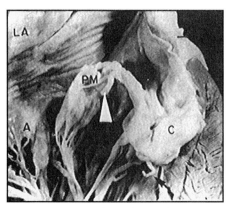

Figure 136: Ruptured chordae serving posteromedial scallop (PM) of the posterior leaflet in a 62-year old man. The scallop has prolapsed prominently. One clubbed, ruptured chorda is in the center (arrow) and a second is at the lower right (arrow).

Clinically, we have found this helpful, although, as might be expected, there are exceptions to this general rule. In some patients there may be combinations of radiation. I used to have some difficulty in remembering which valve caused radiation in which direction. In my naivete, I first thought, "the anterior leaflet — anterior radiation; posterior leaflet — posterior radiation." Now I have no difficulty in remembering that it is opposite to what I first thought!

- **Mitral Regurgitation as a Single Valvular Lesion — If a patient has mitral regurgitation alone, and no other significant findings, you can be almost certain it is *not* of rheumatic etiology as formerly thought, but related to a complication of mitral valve prolapse, such as floppy valve or rupture of a chorda tendinea (Figure 136).**

- **Acute Mitral Regurgitation — The murmur of severe acute mitral regurgitation is loud (grade 4 or above), occupies all of systole, peaks in mid-systole and decreases in the latter part of systole (Figure 137).**

This is typical of chordal rupture, a serious complication of mitral valve prolapse. This murmur often radiates up the anterior chest to the aortic area and at times even into the neck. It may even be accompanied by a systolic thrill over the aortic area. It is easy to appreciate why this condition might be confused with aortic stenosis.

At times differentiation between this complication of mitral valve prolapse and hypertrophic cardiomyopathy has to be considered. Both of these conditions can be remarkably similar. A subtle but very important cardiac pearl:

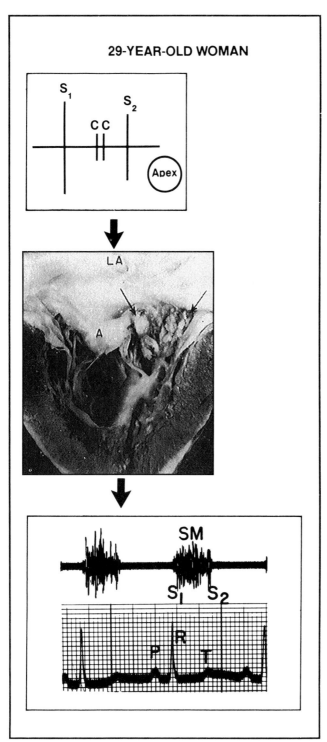

29-YEAR-OLD WOMAN

S₁

S₂

C C

Apex

LA

A

SM

S₁ S₂

P R T

Figure 137: A Female Patient —
Initially the patient had only a couple of midsystolic clicks and no other evidence of heart disease. She was asymptomatic (top panel).

Subsequently she had infective endocarditis (an example shown in another patient — middle panel). The arrows are pointing to the ruptured chordae tendineae.

Although the endocarditis was cured with antibiotics, rupture of a major chordae tendineae had occurred, resulting in acute severe mitral regurgitation (bottom panel). Note the holosystolic murmur of ruptured chordae which characteristically decreases in the latter part of systole.

- **Be sure to pay close attention to the splitting of the second heart sound. Paradoxical splitting (Figure 138) immediately diagnoses hypertrophic cardiomyopathy (in the absence of left bundle branch block, of course, which would be rare).**

- **Women are more likely to have mitral valve regurgitation than men. The reason is unknown.**

Although women have a higher incidence of mitral valve prolapse, men are more likely to have rupture of chordae tendineae, producing mitral regurgitation. Mitral regurgitation is also a cause of wide splitting of the second sound (Figure 139). With systole, blood is ejected through the usual aortic outflow track and simultaneously through the incompetent mitral valve into the left atrium. The left ventricular contents thereby empty earlier than usual, and the aortic valve closure (A_2) is earlier, which results in a wider split in both expiration and inspiration.

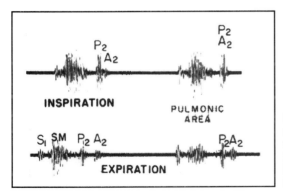

Figure 138: **Splitting** — A patient with paradoxical splitting of the second sound (A_2 - P_2). Note reversed wide split (P_2 - A_2) of second sound with expiration (bottom panel), and close or single split with inspiration (top panel). A systolic murmur (SM) is also present.

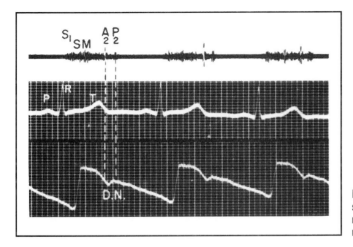

Figure 139: **Wide splitting** of the second sound (A_2 - P_2) with mitral regurgitation. Note holosystolic murmur (SM).

All valvular lesions can, at times, be "silent," with no murmur. The most common silent lesion is mitral stenosis — but in the majority of these, failure to detect a murmur is because the bell of the stethoscope is not over the point of maximal impulse, a localized spot (which may be the size of a quarter) where the diagnostic rumble is heard.

Mitral regurgitation can occasionally be silent and can afford a clue as to malfunction of a prosthetic valve, the sutures of which have become so detached from their insertion that there is severe regurgitant "welling up" of blood with systole — and producing no murmur. Of course when this occurs, cardiac compensation is replaced by severe heart failure, which if promptly recognized might be corrected at surgery.

- **If moderate to severe mitral regurgitation as a *single* valvular lesion is present, the most common etiology is mitral valve prolapse with rupture of a chorda tendinea or floppy valve. It is *not* rheumatic, as was formerly thought.**

Rupture of a chorda tendinea is the most frequent serious complication of mitral valve prolapse. The clinical features of chordal rupture with mitral prolapse vary, depending on the size and/or number. It can occur spontaneously or as a result of infective endocarditis. There are many auscultatory variants of mitral valve prolapse. Any of these, even including a single systolic click, can, with chordal rupture, become a holosystolic murmur of mitral regurgitation. It typically peaks in mid-systole and decreases in the latter part of systole. This configuration of the murmur is due to a significant regurgitant leak of the mitral valve into a normal-sized left atrium, which occurs with chordal rupture; as a pressure in the atrium builds up, it reaches a peak in mid-systole, because the atrium cannot continue to accommodate the large leak, and then the pressure decreases, as does the volume of blood in the last part of systole. The systolic murmur reflects this pressure change.

On the other hand, with chronic significant mitral regurgitation, there is an enlarged left atrium that can continue to accommodate the large volume of blood regurgitating into it.

- **Differentiation between the systolic murmur of aortic stenosis and that of mitral regurgitation — At times it is difficult to differentiate between the murmur of aortic stenosis and that of mitral regurgitation. To do so, listen specifically to the murmur after a pause with a premature beat, or to the beat following a pause with a premature beat, or to the beat following a pause with atrial fibrillation. The**

murmur of aortic stenosis increases in intensity, whereas the murmur of mitral regurgitation shows little change (Figure 140). Utilization of this pearl can make this diagnosis in patients where the differentiation can be extremely difficult. It can even be lifesaving, as it was in the following patient.

A woman of some 60 + years of age was incapacitated because of advanced congestive heart failure. She could not climb even one flight of stairs because of her shortness of breath, and at night had to sleep upright in a chair because of nocturnal dyspnea. She had all of the symptoms and signs of advanced cardiac decompensation. All medications she was taking were not effective in affording relief, and she was considered to have end-stage heart disease.

She stated that she had been told that she had mitral stenosis and regurgitation and atrial fibrillation. On auscultation of her heart, atrial fibrillation was present, and by concentrating on the beat following a pause, there was a definite increase in intensity of the systolic murmur heard over the lower left sternal border and apex. The murmur was not of a harsh quality, but had frequencies that are often heard with that of mitral regurgitation. There was no opening snap of mitral stenosis, but instead an S_3 diastolic gallop. The increase in the systolic murmur following the pause was the clue that this was consistent with aortic stenosis, rather than mitral regurgitation.

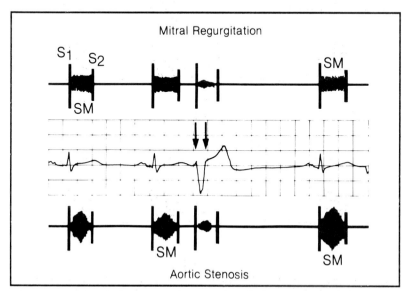

Figure 140: Mitral Regurgitation — Systolic murmur (SM) of mitral regurgitation remains unchanged after pause; in contrast, systolic murmur (SM) of aortic stenosis is louder after pause following premature beat.

The patient had cardiac catheterization following this observation, and she had a gradient over 100 mm across her aortic valve. She then had aortic valve replacement surgery, with a remarkable improvement in her condition to the extent that she was able to return to practically normal physical activities and a comfortable life. She is now approximately nine years following cardiac surgery. In her case, paying attention to the cardiac pearl concerning the increase in the systolic murmur after a pause of atrial fibrillation (or a premature beat) proved to be lifesaving. She had a *reversible* type of heart disease. Such cases are gratifying to the patient, the family, and also to the physician.

The typical holosystolic murmur of significant mitral regurgitation fills all of systole, starting with the first heart sound and continuing to the second sound; sometimes, with more advanced regurgitation, it extends beyond the aortic valve closure (S_2), as some regurgitation continues across the incompetent mitral valve into the left atrium.

- **The holosystolic murmur of mitral regurgitation characteristically decreases coincident with inspiration (in contrast to that of tricuspid regurgitation, which increases (Figure 141).**

It is sometimes said that the systolic murmur of mitral regurgitation "obscures" or "masks" the first heart sound. This is not so, as the first sound can be detected if carefully searched for; the murmur begins with that first sound (Figure 142).

A palpable thrill over the apex indicates mitral regurgitation as well as a grade 4, or above, systolic murmur.

A third heart sound (S_3) is an expected finding in the more advanced, more severe leaks of the mitral valve. A short diastolic rumble may also be heard in such patients. These auscultatory findings are caused by the large volume of blood in the enlarged left atrium filling the ventricle and producing, in the rapid filling phase, the third sound plus low-frequency vibrations. This rumble is usually not the result of stenosis of the mitral valve.

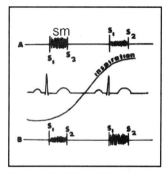

Figure 141: Differential — Note holosystolic murmur (SM) of mitral regurgitation decreases in intensity with inspiration (A); the holosystolic murmur of tricuspid regurgitation increases with inspiration (B).

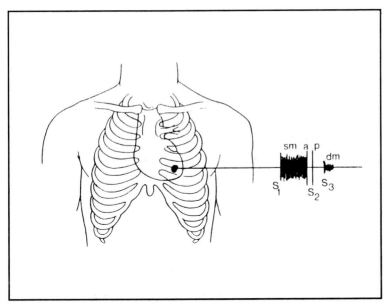

Figure 142: Severe Regurgitation — Findings on auscultation of severe mitral regurgitation: Holosystolic murmur (SM); wider splitting (A-P) of second sound (S₂) (not becoming single with expiration), a third heart sound (S₃) with a short rumble murmur (DM). The first sound (S₁) is not "masked" by the systolic murmur (as some have mistakenly stated).

- **A giant left atrium (large enough to hold a grapefruit or small bowling ball) can be identified on x-ray of the heart and by echo. Cardiac Pearl: Even if a diastolic rumble murmur is present in addition to the typical systolic murmur of mitral regurgitation, the significant and predominant lesion is that of mitral regurgitation.**

Mitral Stenosis

- **If a diastolic rumble of mitral stenosis is present it is almost always heard over the point of maximum impulse of the left ventricle with the patient turned to the left lateral position. Sometimes one has difficulty in palpating this impulse. Check to see if the stethoscope is still in the ear canals. If so, remove it; surprisingly, the spot is often readily felt (Figure 143). This spot may be no larger than a quarter. By removing the stethoscope, which can be a distraction, one can concentrate solely on only one tactile sensation, that of the localized point of maximal impulse.**

Almost always, an opening snap of mitral stenosis is heard, even with the most extensive degrees of stenosis. However, just recently a patient with severe stenosis having a calcified valve "like a rock" did not have an opening snap, nor a loud first sound; instead S_1 was faint, making it even more unusual. "Never say never!" The echocardiogram was most helpful in diagnosis and explanation of the physical findings.

- **The "Trill" of Mitral Stenosis — At our institution what we have termed a "trill" is the presence of three sounds heard over the pulmonic area or third left sternal border at the time of the second heart sound.**

Two of the three components are comprised of the loud, closely split second sound (increased intensity due to the loud pulmonary valve component), followed by another sound, the opening snap of mitral stenosis and heard over the pulmonic area and third left sternal border. On expiration, the splitting of the second heart sound may be close, but still not single. With inspiration, the split widens so that the aortic and pulmonic components are heard even more distinctly, in addition to the opening snap (Figure 144).

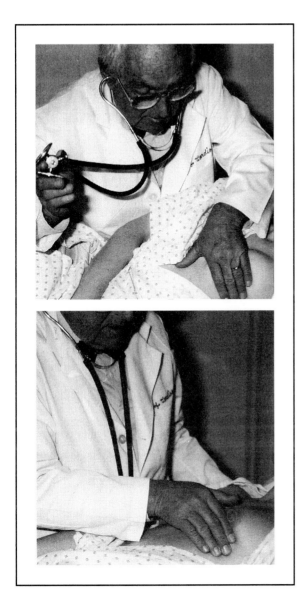

Figure 143: Point of Maximal Impulse — If difficulty is experienced in locating a precordial impulse (top photo), remember that if your stethoscope is still in your ears it can be a distraction; remove it (lower photo). Then note that you now may readily find the impulse. Use the other hand if necessary to better palpate the impulse.

● These three heart sounds or "trill" can be useful in distinguishing mitral stenosis from other conditions. For example, atrial septal defect might be confused with mitral stenosis, particularly if there is atrial fibrillation (more likely in an older patient) and a diastolic rumble which can occur with larger

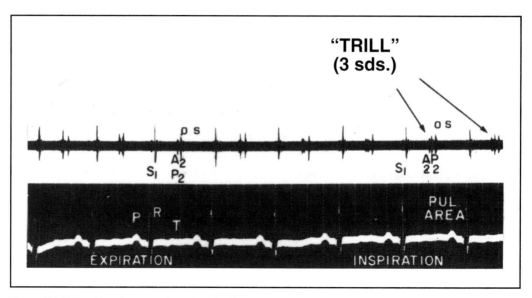

Figure 144: Trill — Note three sounds are heard with inspiration: the aortic (A₂) and pulmonic (P₂) components of the second sound, plus the opening snap (OS) of mitral stenosis. On expiration, only two sounds might be identified (the A₂ and P₂ heard as one sound plus the opening snap as a second sound).

shunts. Differentiating between these two conditions can be difficult, but often can be distinguished by paying attention to the second heart sound. With mitral stenosis, there is a "trill" with three components, whereas with atrial septal defect there are only two components, the aortic and pulmonary valve components. The atrial defect has so-called "fixed" splitting of the second heart sound, whereas mitral stenosis has a more closely split second sound on expiration, widening with inspiration, and followed by the third sound, the opening snap.

I recall two patients from one of our medical conferences; both were ladies in their early 60's who many years ago had been diagnosed as having mitral stenosis. Both had atrial fibrillation; however, they only had two components of the second sound, the wider split of the atrial and pulmonic components and no "trill" (Figure 145). This cardiac pearl enabled the correct diagnosis, atrial septal defect, subsequently proven on cardiac catheterization.

- **Dyspnea — Women are more likely to have a "tight" mitral stenosis than men. Significant dyspnea may occur with sexual intercourse.**

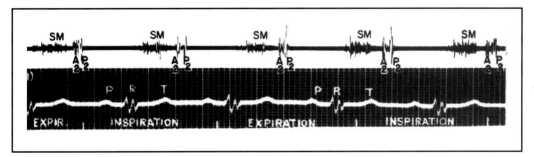

Figure 145: Atrial Septal Defect: Note wide splitting of second sound (A_2 - P_2). There is slight widening of the split with inspiration. There are only two components of S_2, A_2 and P_2 distinguishing it from the "trill" of mitral stenosis, when three sounds may be detected.

In fact, some patients may have acute pulmonary edema precipitated by this act. A physician should ask specifically concerning this because often the patient is reluctant to bring this up without being asked.

- **Loud First Heart Sound** — **If a patient who has a normal heart rate has a loud first sound, always think of two conditions: mitral stenosis and a short P-R interval on the electrocardiogram.**

The length of a P-R interval can affect the first heart sound. The increase in intensity of the sound is most likely due to the position of the atrioventricular (A-V) valves at the time systole occurs. If the valves are deeper in the ventricles and systole occurs promptly after the atrial systole, the valves close, making a louder sound. If the P-R interval is prolonged and the A-V valves have had time to move upward in the ventricles, systolic contraction produces a faint first sound.

A loud first heart sound due to a short P-R interval can simulate the sound of mitral stenosis. The presence of a normal physiologic third heart sound can be misinterpreted as an opening snap.

A young college track star, a long distance runner, had been diagnosed as having mitral stenosis, which, of course, was devastating news to this young person. He was referred to us for consultation; examination showed that he had a short P-R interval, which caused the accentuated first sound, and a normal physiologic third heart sound — misinterpreted as an opening snap. These were normal findings, which made one happy athlete!

In the case of mitral stenosis, an opening snap should be heard and by turning the patient to the left lateral position and listening over the point of maximum impulse of the left ventricle, the telltale diastolic rumble should be present.

If the ventricular heart rate is normal and if the first sound is loud, a short P-R interval or mitral stenosis should be considered.

Graham Steell Murmur (Figure 146) — It has been said that one cannot tell the difference between the diastolic murmur of pulmonary regurgitation (Graham

Steell) associated with mitral stenosis and that of aortic regurgitation associated with mitral stenosis. One *can,* however, make this differentiation. The great majority of patients in which this differentiation must be made will prove to have aortic rather than pulmonic regurgitation.

- **The murmur of aortic regurgitation may be heard over the aortic area and transmitted along the lower left sternal border to the apex. The Graham Steell murmur is not heard over the aortic area and often is localized to the left sternal border and generally not heard at the apex. The peripheral pulse has a quick rise "flip" with aortic regurgitation and not with the Graham Steell murmur.**

Right ventricular hypertrophy can be present with both of them, as noted on electrocardiogram and x-ray, whereas if any degree of left ventricular hypertrophy is present, the patient probably has aortic regurgitation. Echocardiography obviously would aid in this differentiation.

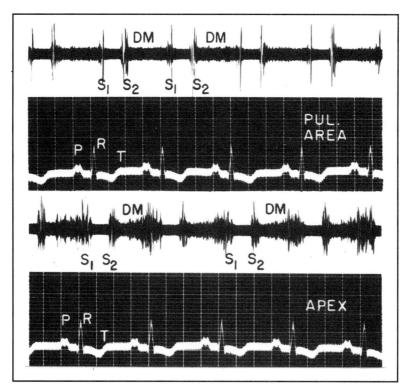

Figure 146: Graham Steell Murmur — Top: Note high frequency diastolic murmur (DM) following an accentuated second sound (S_2); it occupies all of diastole (pulmonic area). At apex the diastolic rumble (DM) occupies all of diastole with presystolic accentuation.

- **Hemoptysis** — **Hemoptysis can occur in the patient having advanced tight mitral stenosis.**

Fortunately, the bleeding, which is due to a rupture of a bronchial vein, is generally self limited and does not represent an emergency situation. However, there have been isolated case reports where the bleeding did not spontaneously subside and surgery was necessary to control it. Pulmonary emboli can also cause hemoptysis with mitral stenosis as well as with other conditions. This can represent a serious complication requiring prompt recognition and treatment.

- **Dyspnea While Swimming** — **A patient with a tight mitral stenosis may experience shortness of breath when getting in a swimming pool or another body of water (lake, ocean) and being immersed up to the neck.**

The shortness of breath may occur without any swimming movements, but be caused simply by the act of being submerged in the water. The mechanism of this would seem to be the fact that there is increased venous return to the heart as the body is being submerged in the water. This cardiac pearl is poorly recognized and one has to ask the patient specifically about this. Dr. Thorpe Ray of New Orleans was, I believe, the first person to make this observation.

- **Dyspnea** — **A patient with a tight mitral stenosis (Figure 147) often develops shortness of breath when sweeping, vacuuming, scrubbing the floor, making the bed, or otherwise working in a stooped position.**

Dyspnea may also occur when climbing even one flight of stairs. On the other hand the patient may be quite comfortable walking on a flat surface, doing her shopping, etc. On stopping the physical activity causing the shortness of breath, the dyspnea may promptly subside.

Differential diagnosis of the opening snap of mitral stenosis and third heart sounds:
1. Exert pressure on the stethoscope, which should eliminate the normal third heart sound or the S_3 (ventricular) diastolic gallop; pressure on the stethoscope is not likely to eliminate the opening snap.
2. The opening snap is heard over the pulmonic area (sometimes aortic area) but not the third sound.
3. The opening snap of a "tight mitral stenosis" is closer to the second sound than the third heart sound.
4. The opening snap serves as a clue to listen over the point of maximal impulse of the left ventricle for the "tell-tale" diastolic rumble — not so with the third sound which does not initiate the diagnostic rumble.

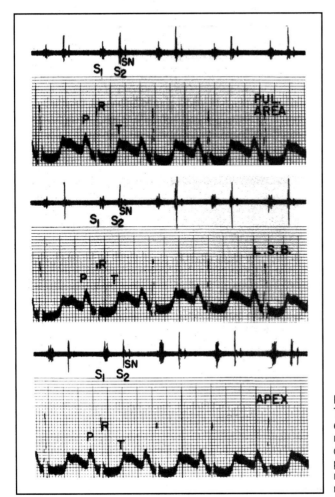

Figure 147: Silent Mitral Stenosis —
This patient had been previously
examined and had a classic diastolic
rumble beginning with the opening snap,
occupying all of diastole and with
presystolic accentuation. Now no diastolic
murmur is present. This patient had a tight
mitral stenosis proved at surgery.

- **The Malar Flush of Mitral Stenosis —**
  The malar flush of mitral stenosis generally
  occurs in patients who have more advanced
  degrees of stenosis. Today this sign is not
  found as frequently as in the past when mitral stenosis was so prevalent. It simulates
  the color of makeup such as "blush" or
  "rouge" over the cheeks.

- **Carcinoid Syndrome** — Another facial
  characteristic that is important is the violaceous hue over the cheeks and face of the
  patient with carcinoid syndrome.

I remember seeing the first patient ever diagnosed with the carcinoid syndrome in the United States (Figure 148). The patient was first diagnosed by General Thomas Mattingly at Walter Reed Army Hospital; she had been examined at Johns Hopkins Hospital by Dr. Helen Taussig. I saw her at a conference at Walter Reed Army Hospital. Her face was a deep purplish color that I had never seen before and her only cardiac finding was a systolic murmur heard over the pulmonic area. This was subsequently documented to be a mild to moderate degree of pulmonic valve stenosis. There was no shunt to explain this particular coloration, which some had believed was cyanosis.

Dr. Mattingly had read an article in one of the cardiology journals describing a new "carcinoid syndrome" described by Dr. Bjork of Scandinavia. Dr. Mattingly thought this particular patient had the features described in this syndrome. By chance, Dr. Bjork was attending the World Congress of Cardiology being held in Washington at that time and the patient was presented to him on rounds at Walter Reed Army Hospital. He agreed that this patient had the carcinoid syndrome. She was therefore the first carcinoid patient diagnosed in the United States; she was then studied by Dr. Al Sjordsma and his colleagues at the National Institutes of Health. They demonstrated the relationship of serotonin in producing features of this syndrome.

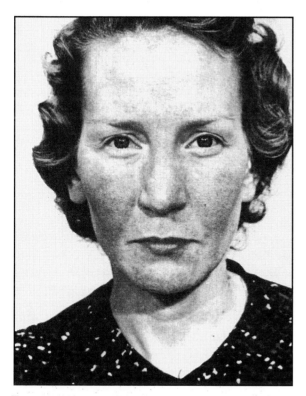

Figure 148: Carcinoid Syndrome — The first patient with carcinoid syndrome diagnosed in the United States. She had a permanent violaceous hue over her face, as shown.

Arrhythmias

The majority of people with normal hearts probably are unaware of an occasional premature beat. Even those having frequent premature beats may not be conscious of them, or may notice only a portion of such beats. I recall, as a young physician, a member of the Harvard crew whom I was asked to evaluate regarding his participating in an upcoming race. He was a well developed, healthy, strapping athlete, the picture of health. He was asymptomatic, and on examination I realized why this evaluation was requested. He had many premature ventricular beats (none occurring in short runs of ventricular tachycardia), although with a basic normal sinus rhythm. To my amazement, he was not aware of these beats. The remainder of his evaluation was normal. He was told to go ahead and participate in the race, which he did, and without any problem.

This patient taught me that a person could be insensitive to an arrhythmia. Of course, many patients do feel irregularity of their heart beat, and promptly report to their physician for advice and treatment. Most people with occasional premature beats do not need medication, only explanation and reassurance. When I have such a patient, who may be anxious and worried, I tell them about my own premature beats, which I have had for over forty years, and relate that I am not worried about these benign beats. Often this suffices as far as their treatment is concerned.

A cardiac pearl to aid in the office or bedside evaluation of a patient's complaint of heart palpitations: **What is palpitation to one patient, is not to others, who describe other sensations or personal interpretations.** The use of one's hand over the precordium can be useful and diagnostic (Figure 149). The hand is moved, for the patient to observe, up and down at a regular rate similar to the heartbeat. A quick beat, followed by a pause, simulates the premature beat. More than one quick beat, two or three or more, can thus be simulated. Bigeminal or trigeminal rhythm is also easily reproduced. The patient may indicate that it was not one of these, but the heart beat was faster. Then the hand can move with a more vigorous and regular motion, stating that this is what may occur if someone has a temporary fright, or a near accident while driving the car; the heart normally speeds up with a normal sinus tachycardia. The patient may then say, "It was faster". Now moving the hand faster, ask the patient to identify the motion as a fast irregular, or a regular one. It is interesting to note that the patient frequently can immediately and correctly identify the irregular motion of atrial fibrillation or the regular motion of paroxysmal atrial tachycardia.

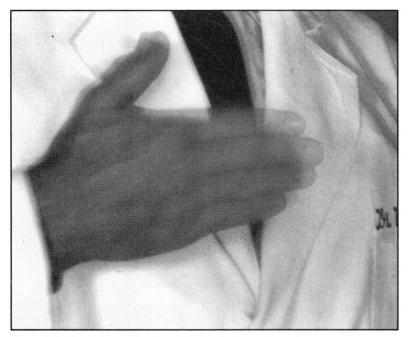

Figure 149: Simulation — Hand in motion simulating a tachycardia.

- **Paroxysmal Atrial Tachycardia — Some patients can have a very rapid ventricular rate of 180 or so and have no symptoms. Others may become dizzy and are immediately aware of the abrupt change in rhythm.**

Called to mind are two patients, one a teenage young lady, the star of her basketball team, who had no heart disease except episodes of paroxysmal atrial tachycardia. Usually she could play competitive basketball without any difficulty, but when this tachycardia occurred she would have to stop. Her tachycardia was well controlled by beta blockers.

Another patient was a lineman for a National Football League team. Occasionally he would have sudden onset of rapid tachycardia and would become dizzy; at that point he would take himself out of the game.

Other patients, however, can have the rapid heart rate of paroxysmal atrial tachycardia without any significant symptoms even during the arrhythmia.

- **Self-Reversion of Paroxysmal Atrial Tachycardia** — Many patients have learned ways to stop their own paroxysmal atrial tachycardia:
  1. Straining, as with a bowel movement.
  2. Placing their hands in ice water and then straining.
  3. Lying on their stomach with their head hanging over the edge of the bed and then straining.
  4. Some patients will stick their finger down their throat to produce gagging, which is sometimes effective.
  5. Some patients have learned that getting into a bathtub of cold water can revert the tachycardia.

I know of one little girl who had mitral valve prolapse and episodes of paroxysmal atrial tachycardia. Her physician learned that if he would hold her by her legs upside down and then produce a sudden jerking movement he could stop her tachycardia. This maneuver was successfully used when she was very young, but of course had to be discontinued when she became a teenager.

- **Paroxysmal Atrial Tachycardia** — The history is that of a sudden onset and cessation of a tachycardia. Rapid, regular ventricular rates of 180 to 200 or above are classic for paroxysmal atrial tachycardia. Carotid sinus pressure, if correctly applied, can, in most patients, result in reversion to normal sinus rhythm (Figures 150A and 150B).

- **Atrial Flutter** — A patient with an untreated atrial flutter having a tachycardia usually has a 2:1 block.

A woman about 30 years of age had returned to her home in the midwest for a holiday; while there she had the onset of a rapid tachycardia and was taken to the emergency room of the local hospital; a drug was administered which caused successful reversion to normal sinus rhythm. On returning home she was referred to me for evaluation. Her description of the tachycardia was corroborated by her watching my moving hands over my chest simulating a very rapid rate of regular rhythm; she said, "yes, it was just like that." This indicated paroxysmal atrial tachycardia. She then showed me the electrocardiogram that had been taken during her tachycardia (which I had been unaware she had possession of) — The computer readout stated that it was atrial flutter. The ventricular rate was 214. A patient on no medication and who had atrial flutter would be 2:1 block; therefore the atrial rate would be 428.

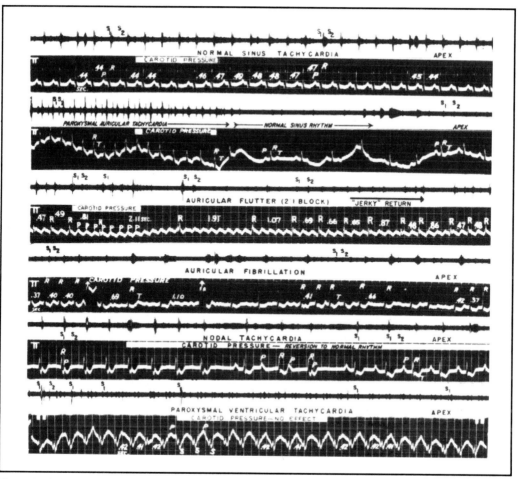

Figure 150A: Composite of Effect of Carotid Sinus Pressure on Various Tachycardias — First tracing: Sinus tachycardia, gradual slight slowing, with smooth return to original normal rhythm. Second tracing: Atrial tachycardia, abruptly stopped, followed by normal rhythm. Third tracing: Atrial flutter. Note prompt slowing of ventricles with irregular "jerky" return to original 2:1 flutter. The atria remain undisturbed. Fourth tracing: Atrial fibrillation. Rate originally irregular and rapid. Immediate slowing with irregular return to former irregular rhythm. Fifth tracing: Nodal tachycardia. Abrupt reversion to normal rhythm (like paroxysmal atrial tachycardia). Sixth tracing: No effect whatsoever on ventricular tachycardia.

- **Atrial flutter is usually between 250 and 350 beats per minute; 428 is too fast for the usual flutter; 214 is consistent with paroxysmal atrial tachycardia. The computer readout was incorrect. This emphasizes that even though most computer interpretations are correct, the "human" electrocardiographer should review the tracings.**

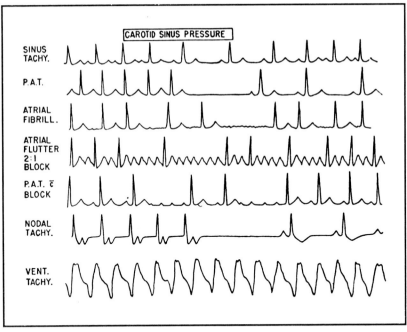

Figure 150B: Composite Artist's Sketch of Effect of Carotid Sinus Pressure on Various Tachycardias. First strip: Note gradual slowing and gradual return to former rate with normal sinus tachycardia. Second strip: Paroxysmal atrial tachycardia (PAT) abruptly stopped, followed by regular rhythm. Third strip: Atrial fibrillation. Rate originally irregular and rapid. Immediate slowing with irregular return to former rhythm. Fourth strip: Note prompt slowing with irregular "jerky" return to original 2:1 flutter. The atria remain undisturbed. Fifth strip: Carotid pressure produces slowing with return to former rate. Note atrial waves easily identified slowing. Sixth strip: Abrupt reversion from nodal rhythm to normal (like paroxysmal atrial tachycardia). Seventh strip: No effect whatsoever on ventricular tachycardia.

- **Another cardiac pearl: In a woman of this age, who never had any previous heart problem and then had sudden onset of an arrhythmia, the diagnosis that should head the differential is mitral valve prolapse.**

    Sure enough, careful examination of this woman revealed typical auscultatory findings, including several systolic clicks, indicative of mitral valve prolapse.

- **Atrial Flutter — Poorly recognized is that atrial flutter can have a change in intensity of the first heart sound. This is shown in Figures 151 and 152.**

    Similar to the fact that a short P-R interval produces a loud first sound and a prolonged P-R interval produces a faint heart sound, so too, with complete heart

176

block, when the independent atrial and ventricular contractions result in a P-wave occurring just before the R wave, the first heart sound is loud; when the P wave is farther from the R wave, the first heart sound is faint. This is what causes the changes in intensity of the first heart sound in complete heart block.

In the same way, if on the electrocardiogram one measures the atrial flutter wave either from the peak of the P wave or from the trough of the flutter waves to the R, or the notching of the downward stroke, there will be a certain "P-R range" in any of these measurements in which the first heart sound in flutter is loud or the reverse, it is on the fainter side.

- **This auscultatory bedside clue can be helpful in suspecting atrial flutter with varying block. This change in intensity of the first heart sound can be even more pronounced with flutter than with atrial fibrillation.**

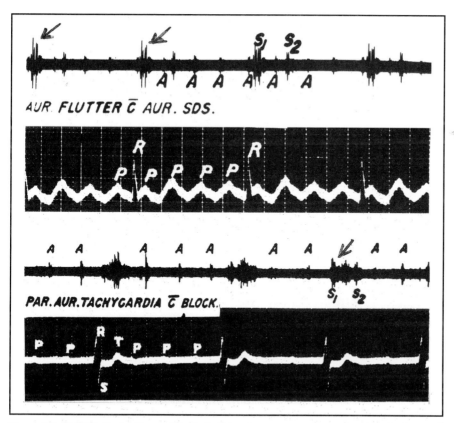

Figure 151: Atrial Flutter — Note atrial sounds (A) and changing intensity of first heart sound with atrial flutter (top tracing) and also paroxysmal atrial tachycardia with block. Louder first sounds indicated by arrows.

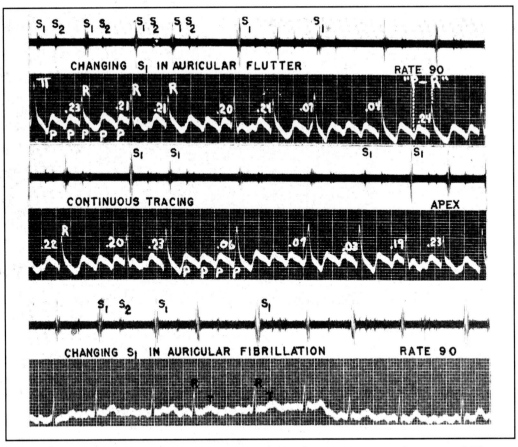

Figure 152: Flutter vs Fibrillation — Note changing first sound (S_1) in upper tracing. Loud S_1 occurs in "P-R" range of .19 to .24 second with loudest at .20 second. Note faint S_1 with fourth and fifth complexes (second strip) which follow longer diastoles; seventh complex shows loud sound with short diastole. Lower tracing shows auricular fibrillation at same rate as above tracing with auricular flutter. The first sounds (S_1) are more constant with auricular fibrillation.

Atrial sounds indicating that atrial contraction is taking place can, at times, also be heard. Flutter waves can also be seen in the jugular venous pulse.

- **Untreated flutter is generally 2:1 block. It may simulate paroxysmal atrial tachycardia. With carotid sinus stimulation, an abrupt slowing may take place, but there is a so-called "jerky" return to the previous rate (Figures 150A and B).**

This is due to the temporary change of the 2:1 block to higher grades of block such as 4:1, 3:1, and so forth and then back to the original regular 2:1 block. Carotid sinus pressure does not cause reversion of the tachycardia to normal sinus rhythm. However, as just noted, carotid sinus stimulation can cause paroxysmal atrial tachycardia to revert to normal sinus rhythm.

178

Ventricular tachycardia can be rapid and might appear to be regular. Actually, however, a very slight irregularity may be present. An important clue is a change in intensity of the first heart sound. In addition, there may be multiple staccato sounds in diastole and sometimes even in systole. Carotid sinus pressure produces no effect. Recognition of this ventricular tachycardia can be lifesaving (Figures 153 and 154).

- **Another pearl worthy of emphasis: Carotid sinus pressure usually has no effect on ventricular tachycardia.**

- **Atrial Fibrillation — The unexplained onset of atrial fibrillation in a patient who is 50 years of age or older may be a clue to the presence of underlying coronary artery disease. However, this is not necessarily true, since other conditions can cause this.**

One example was President Bush's atrial fibrillation, which apparently was triggered by hyperthyroidism. His hyperthyroidism was treated and in turn the atrial fibrillation has apparently been controlled.

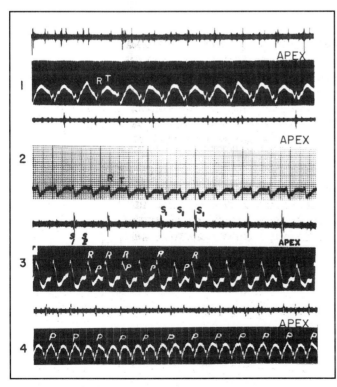

Figure 153: Four patients with ventricular tachycardia showing multiple sounds and a changing intensity of the first sound (S$_1$).

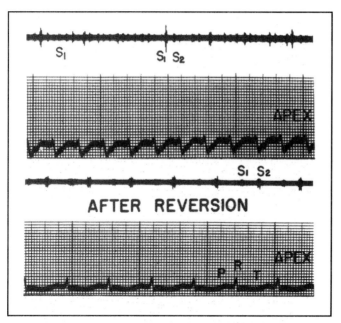

Figure 154: Multiple Sounds — Man, 58 years old, several weeks after acute myocardial infarction. Upper tracing: Ventricular tachycardia showing multiple sounds and changing intensity of first sound (S_1). Lower tracing: Immediately after reversion to normal sinus rhythm. Multiple sounds are absent; first and second sounds are constant, though diminished in intensity.

- **Management of Atrial Fibrillation —** There is still a place for the medical treatment of paroxysmal atrial fibrillation. Too often the first step in management is to have electroconversion, whereas if antiarrhythmic drugs are given under supervision this can be accomplished medically.

    It is best to have the patient under supervision in the hospital when attempting conversion to normal sinus rhythm, either with medication or electroconversion.

- **Multiple Sounds of Ventricular Tachycardia —** This is a poorly recognized but important auscultatory finding of ventricular tachycardia. As noted in Figure 154, there are patients with ventricular tachycardia who have multiple sounds. Note that immediately after reversion, the multiple sounds have disappeared.

No other rhythm is similar to this, and it can be detected at the bedside. However, one must search carefully for this characteristic feature.

- **The presence of an arrhythmia caused by premature beats, either atrial or ventricular, can serve as a predictor of possible tachycardia.**

  For example, frequent atrial premature beats (Figure 155) may be an ominous sign of impending atrial fibrillation.

- **Cardiac Pearl: A patient with mitral stenosis who develops frequent atrial premature contractions is in danger of developing atrial fibrillation.**

  Therefore, it is wise to anticipate this and prescribe a daily anti-arrhythmic as prophylaxis.

  If a patient with known heart disease such as coronary artery disease or cardiomyopathy develops frequent ventricular premature beats, they may be a clue that the subsequent tachycardia will be of the ventricular type.

  Another cardiac pearl: A history of a previous tachycardia is obtained from a patient, but there was no documentation of it. If the patient is having frequent ventricular ectopy, it is likely that the previous tachycardia was of ventricular origin; on the other hand, if atrial premature beats are currently present, then the etiology of the previous tachycardia would likely be of atrial origin — atrial fibrillation or paroxysmal atrial tachycardia.

- **Change of Normal Sinus Rhythm to Atrial Fibrillation — A patient with heart disease may have no evidence of cardiac decompensation, but acute pulmonary edema can occur with the change from normal sinus rhythm to atrial fibrillation. This also may be the first indication of underlying heart disease in some patients.**

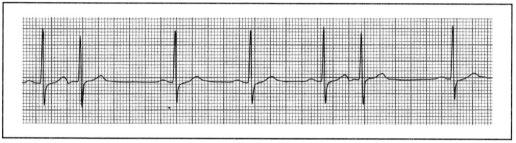

Figure 155: Premature Beats — Tracing from a patient with atrial premature beats occurring every 3-6 beats. He was unaware of these extra beats.

One patient I recall was a 64-year-old woman who was admitted to the Emergency Room of a hospital with acute pulmonary edema, which occurred following the onset of atrial fibrillation. She was given digitalis, but even in increasing doses it did not control her fibrillation. It was realized that, whereas most patient's atrial fibrillation can be slowed with digoxin, hers could not. Verapamil, however, was successful in converting the supraventricular rate to normal, and with quinidine she reverted to normal sinus rhythm. However, after a few days, she changed back into atrial fibrillation. She was again reverted to normal sinus rhythm, but maintenance quinidine did not prevent her atrial fibrillation.

- **Cardiac Pearl: When it is not possible to control atrial fibrillation after trying several antiarrhythmic drugs, it may be best for both physician and patient to "accept" and live with a chronic atrial fibrillation with a ventricular rate in the 60s and 70s. This patient is now nine years since first being evaluated and is getting along satisfactorily despite her chronic cardiac decompensation, and having had a massive myocardial infarction several years ago.**

- **Patients having chronic cardiac decompensation are more likely to have thrombophlebitis, and in turn pulmonary emboli; this may explain why medical treatment is not working. Searching for this possible complication and treatment with anticoagulants can then result in good control of the patient's heart failure.**

The patient just discussed above also had this complication and is on anticoagulant therapy.

- **Increased Diuresis — More common than realized is the fact that patients having rapid tachycardia (such as paroxysmal atrial tachycardia) may have profuse diuresis associated with it.**

I had not been aware of this until the late Paul Wood of London made this observation on some of his patients. One lady prone to episodes of paroxysmal tachycardia had such an urgency for urination with the onset of tachycardia that she would have to stop to urinate while traveling on a bus from her home to the city. She would excrete a voluminous amount of urine. I have found that one does not elicit this history of diuresis with tachycardia unless it is specifically asked about. I have also seen this with rapid atrial fibrillation, although this is not nearly as common as with paroxysmal atrial tachycardia.

It would seem logical to explain this interesting phenomenon as due to the atrial natriuretic factor.

- **Personally observed have been patients with syncope due to ventricular arrhythmias, tachycardia, and/or transient fibrillation, which represent their first indication of a heart problem.**

The cardiac x-ray might be normal in size and silhouette. A careful search for subtle gallops (S_3 and S_4) might reveal their presence, and afford clues to subtle myocarditis or cardiomyopathy.

- **Antiarrhythmic Medications — Remember that antiarrhythmic drugs, although usually very beneficial in prevention of arrhythmias, can also be pro-arrhythmic, and ironically produce the same fatal arrhythmia that one is trying to prevent.**

Therefore, careful observation and follow-up after initiation of a new antiarrhythmic drug is essential. The possibility of a pro-arrhythmia effect of a drug is not appreciated as well as it should be.

The following is a case in point, which I only learned about recently:

A friend, who is in his late 70s, developed atrial fibrillation. He was anticoagulated as a precaution to prevent emboli coincident or following reversion to normal sinus rhythm. Wisely, he was admitted to the hospital for attempt at medical conversion with quinidine before resorting to electroconversion. On quinidine, he is reported to have developed "torsades des points" ventricular arrhythmia and cardiac arrest (Figure 156). Fortunately he was immediately and successfully resuscitated.

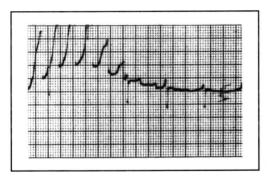

Figure 156: Torsades des points.

Attempts at reversion with either medication or electroconversion are best done in a hospital or a medical facility having trained personnel and equipment to deal with any untoward complication.

- **Slow Ventricular Rate — If on examining a patient you note normal sinus rhythm with a slow ventricular rate such as in the 50s or 60s, think of two things: One, the patient is in good physical training and has developed a slow rate from vagal tone; or two, that the patient might be on a beta blocker.**

For instance, one might examine a person aged 55 or so, and find that he has a healthy slow ventricular rate. You might say, "Are you in any athletic or physical conditioning program such as swimming, playing tennis, or jogging at this time?" And he says, "No." "Are you on a beta blocker?" Again, the answer is "no." Then you might ask, "Were you ever active in athletics?" and the patient may say, "Oh yes, I used to run the mile when I was on the track team in college;" or mention previous participation in some other sport. It is interesting that the vagal tone that is responsible for this development of a slow rate in athletic training when a person was younger, may still persist at a later age in some patients.

- **Cardiac pearl: Remember to deliver a good "thump" on the chest with the clenched fist as an early, initial attempt at treatment of cardiac arrest.**

This chest blow may disturb the fatal ventricular arrhythmia, and convert it into normal sinus rhythm. If not successful, of course, standard cardiopulmonary resuscitation techniques should be promptly given.

However, remember that, occasionally, a chest thump can do the opposite — cause ventricular tachycardia and/or fibrillation.

Death from Fright — "Voo-Doo Death"

I had the opportunity to document a short run of ventricular tachycardia (Figure 157) resulting from fright in a 28-year-old woman who had no heart disease. This brings up the truth of the old expression "scared to death". Having observed this, I went to the Department of Physiology at the Harvard Medical School and inquired if there was any medical publication that I could read on the subject. I was told that the late Dr. Walter Cannon, a renowned Harvard professor of physiology who had just retired, had written an article on voo-doo death. Dr. Cannon apparently believed there was medical credence to some of the reported deaths.

I recall a patient in the intensive care unit of our hospital who was on constant monitoring of his heart beat. As I was watching his monitor at the nurse's station, he had a sudden burst of ventricular tachycardia. I rushed to his room and fortunately the ventricular tachycardia had spontaneously reverted to normal rhythm. He was holding a telephone and was engaged in a heated argument with his daughter, which apparently precipitated the arrhythmia, which could have been fatal. Pleasurable emotions can also trigger arrhythmias, as can stress, tension states and strenuous physical activity.

I remember one patient who had first degree heart block and hypertension associated with a test examination. He was a fourth year medical student who was rejected for a Navy internship because of an elevation of blood pressure and first degree block. He was told, however, that if we could document on three successive days normal findings of the ECG and blood pressure, he would be accepted. He was.

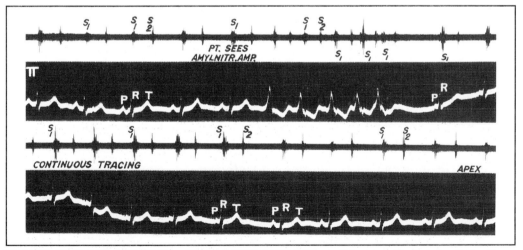

Figure 157: Tachycardia from Fright — An ampule pearl of amyl nitrite was to be inhaled to study its effect on the heart sounds of this patient with a normal heart. On seeing the ampule, the patient became obviously frightened, producing tachycardia, as shown here.

Carotid Sinus Pressure

- **Technique — Carotid sinus stimulation (or pressure) is still a very useful maneuver that can be performed in the office or at the bedside. The technique of performing carotid sinus pressure is shown in Figures 158 and 159.**

    The physician's stethoscope is placed over the precordium to monitor any change in rhythm. (One does not have to hold the stethoscope.) The patient's head is positioned over the physician's left arm. The head is turned to the left and the carotid artery is palpated at the angle of the right jaw. This is where the carotid sinus is located. Press this area with your index and middle finger (some physicians prefer to use their thumb) and feel for the carotid pulsation. Stop the pressure immediately if a response is obtained. If available, the electrocardiogram should be recording the procedure. Remember not to use prolonged carotid sinus stimulation, since serious consequences can occur, such as prolonged cardiac asystole, and even death. Instead press over the carotid sinus for 3 to 5 seconds, then let up for 5 to 10 seconds. Repeat this several times.

- **It is necessary to apply sufficient pressure that it will usually cause some discomfort to the patient.**

- **When carotid sinus pressure is not effective, it usually means that the exact spot of the carotid arterial pulsation at the angle of the jaw has not been located.**

    Caution: Advise the patient not to try "self" carotid sinus pressure.

- **If the patient has a rapid tachycardia, slowing of the ventricular rate with carotid sinus pressure rules out the most serious of arrhythmias, that of ventricular tachycardia.**

- **Precautions — Do not use carotid sinus pressure in a patient who has known cerebral vascular disease.**

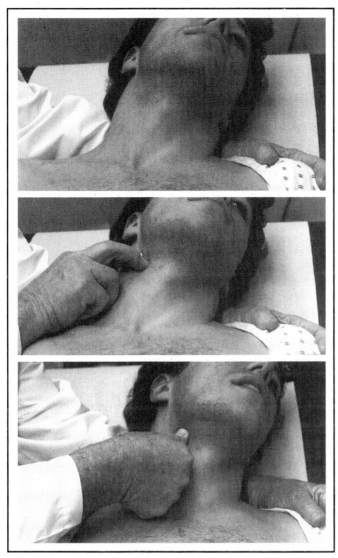

Figure 158: Carotid Sinus Pressure — Remove the pillow and position the patient's head over the your left arm (top). Locate the carotid artery pulsation just under the angle of the right jaw. Exert pressure with the index and middle fingers or thumb. Listen with your stethoscope resting over the precordium (no hand is necessary to hold the stethoscope in place).

The temporary cessation of blood flow resulting from the carotid sinus pressure can decrease cerebral blood flow to the point of causing convulsions and even a stroke. Personally observed was a patient who had convulsions following carotid sinus pressure; fortunately this did not result in any permanent damage.

- **Do not use simultaneous carotid sinus pressure over both right and left sides of the neck.**

- **Even though pressure over the eyeballs has been used and advocated as vagus nerve stimulation in the past, don't use it. Serious injury to the eye can and has resulted.**

- **Carotid sinus hypersensitivity has been noted in some patients with advanced aortic stenosis.**

Hypersensitive carotid sinuses do exist, but are not common. However, such a possibility should be ruled out to avoid serious complications such as asystole and ventricular arrhythmias that can result from carotid sinus pressure.

Make sure there is no abnormality of the carotid arteries, as might be signalled by the finding of significant bruits over either of the carotids. History of previous transient ischemic attack (TIA) or stroke also would contraindicate carotid artery stimulation. If there is no significant change in carotid pulsation or presence of a bruit, place the stethoscope over the chest to monitor any change in the rhythm. (The stethoscope can be positioned so that both hands are free); then while listening with the stethoscope, very gently *touch* the area for carotid sinus stimulation to make sure it is not a hypersensitive carotid sinus.

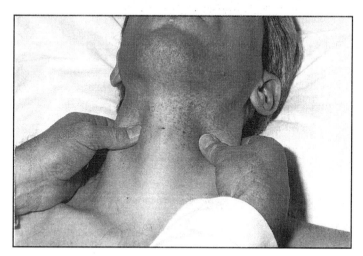

Figure 159: Simultaneous Palpation of Both Carotids — Inequality of pulses can thus be recognized. Caution: Before applying this bilateral palpation, first listen over each carotid to detect any significant murmurs (bruits) of significant arterial obstruction. Also, before palpating as shown above, gently palpate one carotid at a time to rule out a hypersensitive carotid sinus. Caution: Do not apply carotid sinus pressure simultaneously on both sides.

- **A patient with a hypersensitive carotid sinus may show striking, prompt slowing even with this initial gentle palpation.**

A 47-year-old man was evaluated in the office because of a syncopal episode, and the patient's concern that he had heart disease. Pertinent findings from history: While shaving, he stated "everything went blank." He was found on the floor by his wife shortly after this. Apparently he remained "unconscious" for one or one and one half minutes. Profuse perspiration was present. He was then hospitalized at Georgetown University Hospital. Carotid arteriogram was normal. He was seen by neurology and neurosurgical consultants. No intracranial or vascular lesion was demonstrated. He was discharged with the final diagnosis of postural hypotension.

Because the patient believed he had heart disease, he was referred for evaluation. There was no previous history of cardiovascular disease. Physical exam was normal except for the following interesting finding: Remembering from the history that the patient's syncopal episode occurred while shaving, gentle carotid sinus pressure was applied on the right side (the same position of the razor blade when syncope occurred). There was prompt slowing. A wooden tongue blade simulating the razor when shaving was applied over the right carotid sinus area, again resulting in abrupt slowing, as shown in Figure 160. Diagnosis: Hypersensitive carotid sinus.

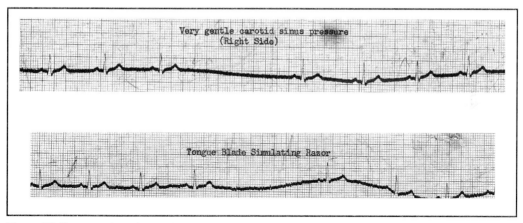

Figure 160: Hypersensitive Carotid Sinus — Upper tracing: Prompt slowing with very gentle carotid sinus pressure. Lower tracing: Similar slowing with pressure over same area with a tongue blade.

Heart Block

When the P-R interval on the ECG is short, the first heart sound may be loud. On the other hand, in the same patient, when the P-R interval is prolonged (such as in first degree heart block) the first heart sound may be faint. The intensity of the first heart sound will relate to the length of the P-R interval (Figures 161 and 162).

- **A slow ventricular heart rate plus a changing intensity of the first heart sound indicates complete heart block.**

In complete heart block, wherein the atrial rate is independent of the ventricular rate, there are multiple opportunities for a change in the relation of the P-wave to the QRS complex. Therefore, when the P is close to the first heart sound, it may be loud. On the other hand, when it is not close and the P-R interval is prolonged and at a distance away from the first heart sound, the sound may be faint. This results in a changing intensity of the first heart sound; at intervals, when the P-R interval is short, an abrupt loud first sound (the "bruit de canon" or "cannon shot") occurs which is an auscultatory finding diagnostic of complete heart block (Figure 163).

Of course, if the ventricular rate is slow, about 40 beats per minute, an early to midsystolic murmur is usually present and in addition, atrial sounds may be heard in diastole, if searched for.

- **Cannon Wave of the Jugular Venous Pulse — The diagnosis of complete heart block can be suspected by paying attention to the jugular venous pulsations in the neck and by observing a slow regular heart rate (approximately 40 beats per minute). If a sudden "cannon wave" occurs, it indicates that atrial contraction is occurring simultaneously with ventricular contraction. This is common with complete heart block.**

If one placed a ping pong ball over the right supraclavicular fossa, the cannon wave might well knock it off.

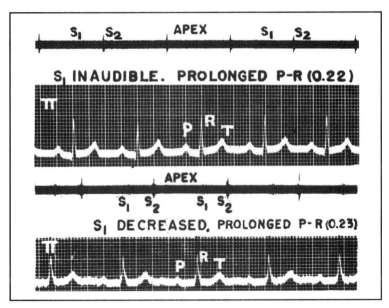

Figure 161: Two Cases of First Degree Heart Block — Note decreased first sound and prolonged P-R interval.

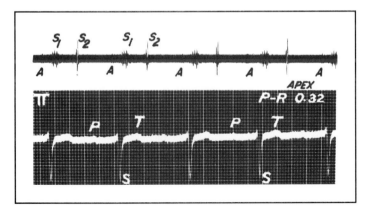

Figure 162: First Degree Heart Block — There is a faint first sound and a fourth sound is heard in presystole; the heart rate is normal.

● **It is a misconception that in complete heart block the loud first heart sound (the so-called "bruit de canon" or cannon shot) occurs at the same time as the cannon wave in the jugular venous pulse. This is incorrect.**

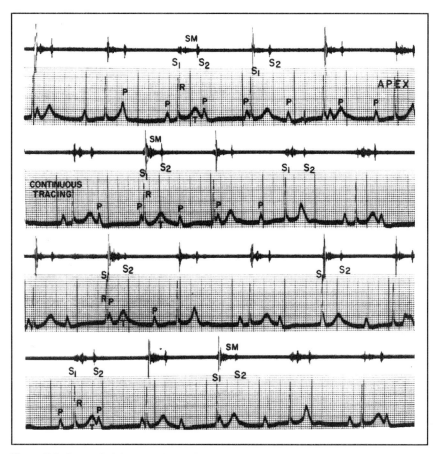

Figure 163: Congenital Complete Heart Block — Note slow heart rate and changing intensity of the first heart sound (S₁). When the P-R interval is short, the first sound is loud; when the P-R interval is prolonged, the first sound is faint. Note short, insignificant systolic murmur (SM).

The loud auscultatory sound has no relation to the cannon wave of the jugular venous pulse. However, they may occur simultaneously if the P-R interval is short enough to produce a loud first sound, and the next P-wave (atrial contraction) occurs with ventricular systole.

- **Palpation of Atrial Contractions in the Arterial Pulse — Complete heart block (in addition to causing a change in intensity of the first sound, atrial sounds heard in diastole, and the visual "cannon waves" in the neck) can also cause faint arterial pulsations which relate to atrial contraction. This represents a seldom recognized physical finding.**

192

Palpation of the radial, brachial, carotid or femoral arterial pulses can identify a pulsation that is coincident with the atrial contraction of diastole. It is interesting that this is a faint but definite arterial pulsation, indicating that the atrial contraction is producing a wave traversing the left ventricle and aortic valve in order to be palpated at the arterial pulse.

- **Intensity of the first heart sound correlating with the length of the P-R interval — With practice, one can become expert in predicting the P-R interval of the electrocardiogram by merely paying attention to the intensity of the first heart sound.**

   A short P-R interval (0.14-0.16 sec) equals a loud first sound. P-R interval of 0.17-0.18 sec equals average intensity. P-R interval of 0.20-0.24 equals faint.

   You can train yourself by jotting down the estimation of the P-R interval from auscultation of the heart, and then compare it with the actual reading on the electrocardiogram. Before too long, one's estimation at the bedside will probably come within two hundredths of a second of the correct P-R interval, provided the patient is of normal body build. An emphysematous or very obese chest would decrease the intensity of the first sound, and a very thin chest, such as a child's, would bring the stethoscope closer to the heart, thereby increasing the intensity of the sound.

   One has to interpolate these variances of the chest configuration; for the obese or emphysematous chest, subtract the estimation of the P-R interval (e.g., if it sounds on the fainter side, 0.19 sec., a normal chest might be estimated at 0.17 sec; with a thin chest, when the sounds are more readily heard, add a little) e.g., 0.14 sec. might become 0.16 sec.

- **Differentiating between normal sinus bradycardia, 2:1 heart block, and complete heart block**

   Figures 164 through 166 show three patients each with a slow heart rate in whom the physician would have to differentiate between normal sinus bradycardia, 2:1 heart block, and complete heart block.

- **With normal sinus bradycardia (Figure 164), the first sound remains constant, no atrial sounds are heard in diastole, and carotid sinus pressure can cause a prompt slowing of the rate.**

   2:1 heart block has a constant first sound and a prominent sound in diastole caused by the atrial contraction coinciding with the normal rapid filling phase (S$_3$) of ventricular diastole (Figure 165).

With complete heart block, there is a changing intensity of the first heart sound, and atrial sounds may be heard in diastole (Figure 166).

Carotid sinus pressure in both the 2:1 heart block and complete heart block may yield no effect, but this is variable.

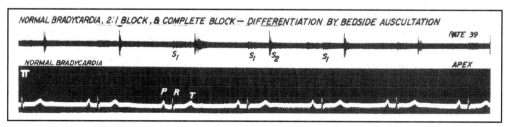

Figure 164: Normal Bradycardia – This tracing is from a 33-year-old woman with no heart disease. The first sound (S_1) remains constant.

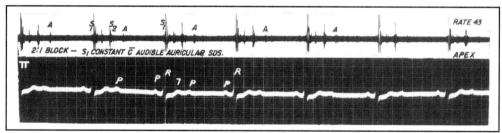

Figure 165: 2:1 Block – This tracing is from a 71-year-old woman with hypertensive heart disease. The rate is slow, S_1 does not vary in intensity, but the atrial sound (A) is heard in early diastole.

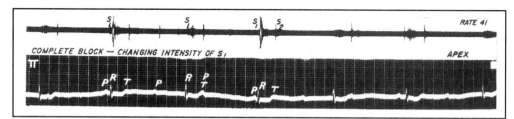

Figure 166: Complete Block – This tracing is from an 80-year-old man with coronary artery disease and transient complete heart block. Note the slow regular rate with marked changing intensity of the first sound (loud S_1 with short P-R). In all three of the above tracings, the ventricular rate is approximately 40.

- **First Degree Heart Block and Dizziness** — A patient having first degree heart block may at times have unexplained dizziness or near syncope. The dizziness may be related to a temporary change from first degree block to 2:1 or complete block.

  It is during this change that the symptoms may occur. Dizziness is unlikely to occur when the block is a constant 2:1, first degree, or complete block.

- **One would think that a patient having the Wolff-Parkinson-White syndrome with a short P-R interval would have a loud first heart sound; however, it is usually of normal intensity.**

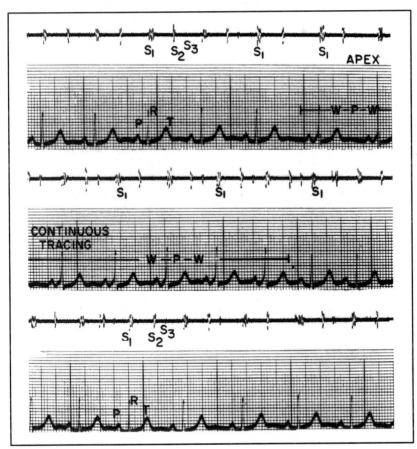

Figure 167: Wolff-Parkinson-White — A 24-year-old woman with Wolff-Parkinson-White Syndrome. The conduction varied between normal and WPW. Note little change in the first sound (S₁).

The shortening of the P-R interval is at the expense of the wide QRS, so the total time from the onset of the P-wave to the end of the QRS is about normal. The right ventricle is stimulated early and the left ventricle response is on time. Figure 167 shows the transition from normal conduction to W-P-W and back to normal. The first sound shows little change.

A historical note concerning Wolff-Parkinson-White: This syndrome of a short P-R interval, wide QRS and episodes of a supraventricular tachycardia has resulted in worldwide interest and I would guess has produced the most voluminous medical literature in the world.

Dr. Louis Wolff of Boston and Sir John Parkinson of London had apparently independently observed these patients. Dr. Paul Dudley White of Boston (Figure 168) was instrumental in putting the records of these patients together and arranging for their publication. The syndrome was, therefore, reported in the medical literature introducing what became known as the Wolff-Parkinson-White Syndrome. Drs. White and Wolff, being in the same city, knew each other. Dr. White also knew Dr. Parkinson but Dr. Wolff did not. It was not until following the Second World Congress of Cardiology held in 1950 (Washington, D.C.) that Dr. White introduced Dr. Wolff to Dr. Parkinson (Figure 169).

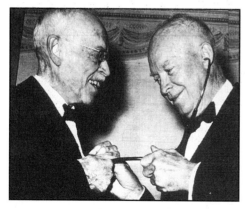

Figure 168: Reverse Roles — President Dwight Eisenhower listening to Dr. Paul Dudley White.

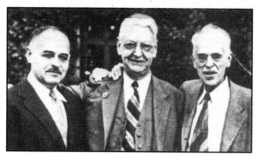

Figure 169: Drs. Wolff, Parkinson and White of the Wolff-Parkinson-White syndrome — Dr. White introduced Dr. Wolff to Dr. Parkinson in Boston. Dr. Parkinson had just attended the Second World Congress of Cardiology (Washington, DC 1950) and he visited Dr. White in Boston at the Massachusetts General Hospital.

Physical Examination

When starting to palpate the precordium on physical examination, it is suggested that the examiner use both hands as shown in Figure 170, which enables the observer to feel both the left side as well as the right side. In this way, one should not overlook dextrocardia (provided the patient is of normal build, not greatly obese, and not having an increase in AP diameter of the chest, as with obstructive emphysema).

Also using both hands, the right hand is placed over the apex of the left ventricle and the other over the aortic area. A left ventricular impulse indicating hypertrophy of the left ventricle can be felt, and a palpable systolic thrill may be noted over the aortic area, the direction of which is towards the right neck and right shoulder. Cardiac pearl relating to the palpable thrill: The direction of the thrill with aortic stenosis is towards the right neck or clavicle. The palpable thrill of pulmonary valve stenosis is toward the left neck and left clavicle.

- **The detection of a palpable thrill, which is easily identified if searched for, means that an aortic systolic murmur at least of grade 4 intensity will be heard; therefore, the patient has aortic stenosis, which is diagnosed by palpation.**

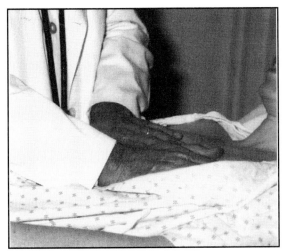

Figure 170: Palpate with Both Hands — In a patient with a normal sized chest, dextrocardia might be immediately detected.

As mentioned previously, when greeting the patient initially and checking the radial pulse, note whether there is a slow rise and a slow descent; if present, this is consistent with aortic stenosis. If there was no quick rise or "flip" of the pulse, one can be sure that there is no significant degree of aortic regurgitation. Therefore the diagnosis from palpation is that of a significant aortic stenosis, with little or no aortic regurgitation. Many times patients undergo a complete workup in the hospital, including even cardiac catheterization, to confirm this diagnosis, which can be made by simple palpation.

- **Although both valvular aortic stenosis and hypertrophic cardiomyopathy can, with the more severe degrees of obstruction, produce paradoxical (or reversed) splitting of the second sound, it is much more common in patients with hypertrophic cardiomyopathy.**

- **Impulses of Hypertrophy — When palpating the left sternal border and apical regions, a systolic impulse felt along the lower left sternal border is consistent with right ventricular hypertrophy. An impulse felt laterally over the apical area is due to left ventricular enlargement and/or hypertrophy. Impulses palpated in the middle, between these two areas, are most likely related to ischemic heart disease (Figure 171).**

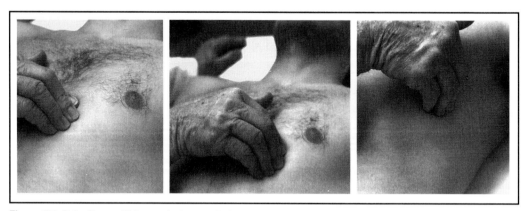

Figure 171: Palpation — Right ventricular systolic impulse (left photo); systolic impulse in between (middle photo) — More likely related to coronary heart disease (ventricular aneurysm, akinesia, dyskinesia of the left ventricle). Left ventricular systolic impulse is shown in the photo on the right.

For example, a left ventricular aneurysm resulting from a previous myocardial infarction may produce a paradoxical systolic bulge with systole as the other areas of the left ventricle are contracting inward. In such circumstances, the electrocardiogram may show another diagnostic clue: Persistent elevation of the S-T segments in the left precordial leads. The combination of this impulse plus the persistent electrocardiographic findings (in the absence of an acute infarction where the same findings may be present) indicates left ventricular aneurysm, most likely due to an old myocardial infarction. At times, this paradoxical systolic bulging impulse can be seen as well as felt.

Physical Examination of the Abdomen

- **Percussion** — **Percussion of the abdomen is a very important part of the physical examination that too often is not performed.**

     Starting at the right lower abdomen and percussing upward, an area of dullness is encountered which indicates the lower edge of the liver (Figure 172). A gentle balloting with the fingers over this area may accurately identify this lower border. The normal liver dullness does not usually extend below the right costal margin. Remember, also, to percuss the upper border of the liver to make sure a normal sized liver has not been displaced downward. I have been told that when actual patients were used in the "practical" part of the cardiology subspecialty Board examinations, one examiner always noted whether both the upper and lower borders of the liver were percussed; if so, it made a favorable impression on that examiner. This percussion technique can also be used in identifying splenic enlargement, aneurysm, or other abdominal mass.

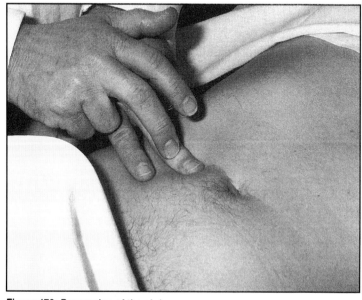

Figure 172: Percussion of the abdomen.

- **Occasionally a patient is hypersensitive (unusually ticklish) about having the examiner percuss (or palpate) over the abdomen. Pearl: The patient can place his or her hand on the abdomen, and percussion can be performed over the patient's hand (Figure 173).**

- **Abdominal Auscultation — Listen to the abdomen of every patient being examined. The bell of the stethoscope is best, using firm pressure to indent the abdomen (Figure 174).**

A faint, short, midsystolic murmur, grade 1 to 3, may be a normal finding over the mid-abdomen and over the aortic pulsation. Systolic murmur (bruits) longer in duration may be a clue to arterial obstruction, as is the case with carotid bruits in the neck. A continuous murmur may indicate an arteriovenous fistula (Figure 175).

Also listen with the bell of the stethoscope over each femoral artery (Figure 176). If you hear a "pistol shot" ejection sound, suspect aortic regurgitation. Pressure over the femoral artery with the bell of the stethoscope may also detect a systolic murmur and a higher frequency diastolic murmur (Duroziez's Sign).

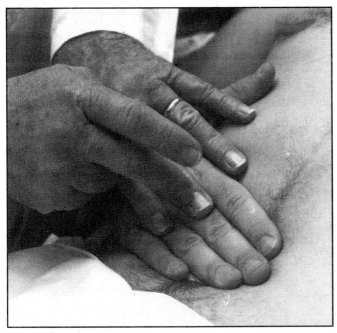

Figure 173: Unusual Percussion — For the patient who is hypersensitive to the physician's percussion, have the patient place his or her hand over the abdomen, and percuss over it. It works!

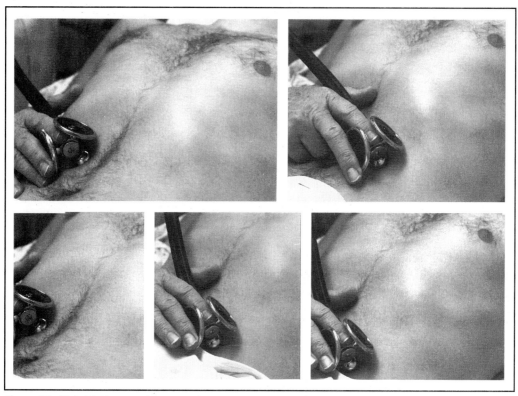

Figure 174: Abdominal auscultation should be done on every patient. Use the bell of the stethoscope.

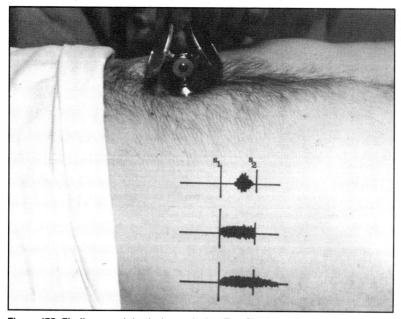

Figure 175: Findings on abdominal auscultation. Top: Short systolic murmur —
May be a normal finding. Middle: Systolic murmur occupies all of systole. Bottom: Continuous murmur.

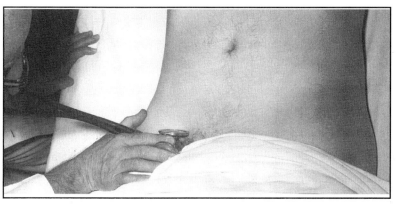

Figure 176: Auscultation of the Femoral Artery — Listening with the bell of the stethoscope over the femoral artery can detect a long systolic murmur (bruit) indicating arterial occlusive disease. If a high frequency diastolic murmur is heard, along with a systolic ejection sound ("pistol shot"), it is a sign of advanced aortic regurgitation.

- **Palpation — It is important to palpate over the base of the heart, as shown in Figure 177.**

     The palpating hand can feel:
     A loud pulmonic valve closure of P_2.
     A systolic ejection sound.
     A systolic thrill of pulmonic valve stenosis.
     A right ventricular lift with the bottom (heel) of the palm.
     A loud aortic valve closure of A_2.
     An aortic systolic ejection sound.
     A systolic thrill of aortic stenosis.
     A diastolic thrill of aortic regurgitation.

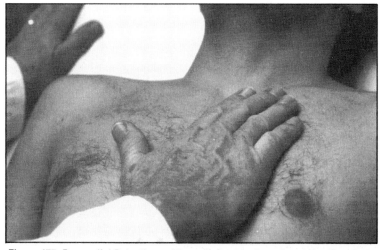

Figure 177: Precordial Palpation — The palpating hand, as shown above, gathers valuable information from the base of the heart and the right and left sternal borders.

- **Abnormal Systolic Pulsations** — If a patient has a systolic pulsation at the sternal end of the right clavicle over the aortic area, is there any normal pulsation that can cause this? No, this is most likely related to aneurysm and/or dissection of the ascending aorta (Figure 178).

- **Palpation with Two Hands** — In addition to detecting dextrocardia (Figure 179), the use of both hands during palpation is helpful in detecting significant mitral regurgitation.

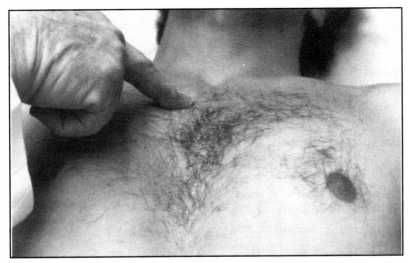

Figure 178: Palpation of a systolic impulse of the sternal end of the right clavicle. This can be caused by aneurysm or dissection of the ascending aorta.

If the right hand is placed over the apex one may feel an impulse in systole indicative of left ventricular hypertrophy; the left hand is placed over the lower left sternal border and if a delayed systolic impulse is felt (Figure 179), this usually indicates an advanced degree of mitral regurgitation into an enlarged left atrium. With systole, which produces the left ventricular impulse, the left ventricular contents are emptied into the large left atrium, which then impinges on the spine, and a "bank shot" results, with the heart being moved forward, producing the delayed impulse along the right sternal border. This is a useful but poorly appreciated and seldom employed cardiac pearl.

If only the area along the lower left sternal border was palpated, then a misdiagnosis of right ventricular hypertrophy would be made. By using both hands and getting a delayed impulse, you will avoid this "trap." It is true, of course, that some patients with mitral regurgitation develop right ventricular hypertrophy. This is caused by the regurgitant mitral leak extending up into the pulmonary veins, eventually resulting in increased pressure on the pulmonary circuit, and in turn, right ventricular hypertrophy. When hypertrophy of the right ventricle is also present, then palpation with both hands reveals that the impulse is not delayed, but rather occurs simultaneously with the left ventricular impulse.

- **Mitral Stenosis** — **A patient who has a tight mitral stenosis with a loud first sound, prominent second sound, opening snap, and diastolic rumble with presystolic accentuation can have palpatory counterparts that can be detected by placing the palm of the hand over the point of maximum impulse of the left ventricle (Figure 180).**

The loud first heart sound is easily felt, as are the vibrations of the accentuated second sound, opening snap, and then the palpable diastolic thrill of the rumble. There is practically no other condition that simulates these specific findings of mitral stenosis.

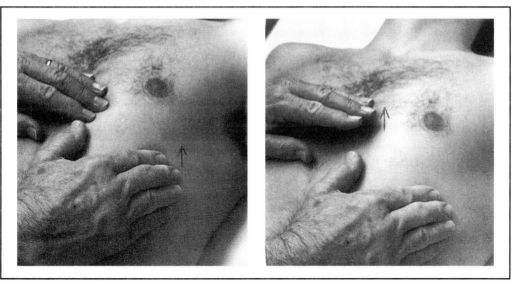

Figure 179: Two-Hand Palpation — Palpation using two hands can help make the diagnosis of significant chronic mitral regurgitation. The left hand palpates an impulse over the lower left sternal border (photo on left). The right hand is over the apex, palpating a left ventricular impulse. A systolic impulse is felt first at the apex (left photo) and then a *delayed* impulse is felt along the lower left sternal border (right photo). Note outward impulse depicted by fingers off chest (arrow).

• One sense at a time.

If difficulty is experienced in locating the point of maximal impulse of the left ventricle with the patient turned to the left lateral position, remember to remove the ear pieces of the stethoscope from the ear canals. The impulse, often the size of a quarter, may then be promptly found. We need to concentrate on one sense at a time; removing the ear tips enables specific single concentration on the sense of touch over the chest wall.

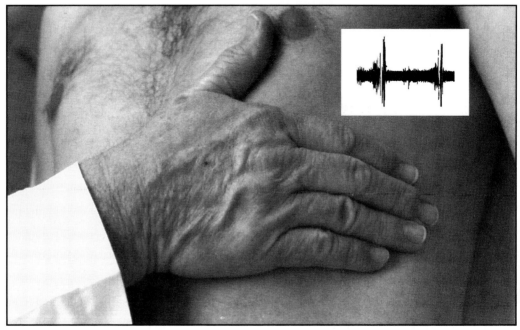

Figure 180: Feeling Stenosis — With a "tight" mitral stenosis, the loud first heart sound, second sound, and opening snap can be palpated, as can the diastolic rumble occupying all of diastole with presystolic accentuation, which produces a palpable diastolic thrill.

The Examining Room

- **The room should be quiet. Acoustic tile on the ceiling (and walls) can help, as can drapes over windows, carpet on the floor, isolation from outside conversation, telephones, loud noisy air conditioning, and typewriters (Figures 181 and 182).**

    Do not attempt to examine a patient who is still clothed. An examining table or bed is necessary so that the patient can be effectively examined in various positions such as lying flat and turned to the left lateral position. Abdominal exam has to be done with the patient lying on his back. Also examine the patient in sitting, standing, and squatting positions.

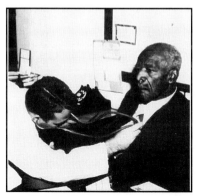 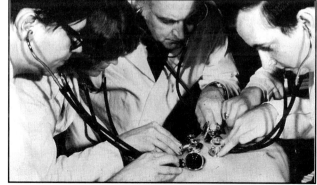

Figures 181 and 182: How not to examine a patient.

- **A simple point, but sometimes overlooked: Make sure the door of the examining room is fully closed.**
- **Ideally, a footstool for use by both the patient and the physician should be in the examining room (Figure 183).**

The patient often needs it to get up and down on the examining table. When listening to the patient in the left lateral position, the physician frequently needs the stool in order to be comfortable and accurately listen — this is particularly apropos for the physician of average or shorter height, when examining a large and/or overweight patient.

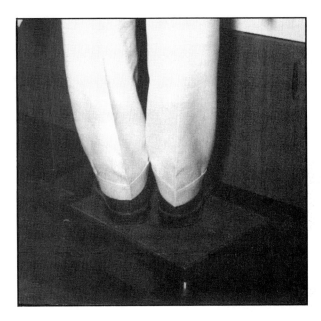

Figure 183: A footstool has frequent use in the examining room for both the physician and the patient.

Physical Exam — Blood Pressure

- **When taking the patient's blood pressure, either in the sitting or lying position, be sure to locate the brachial arterial pulsation and listen with the stethoscope over this area (Figure 184).**

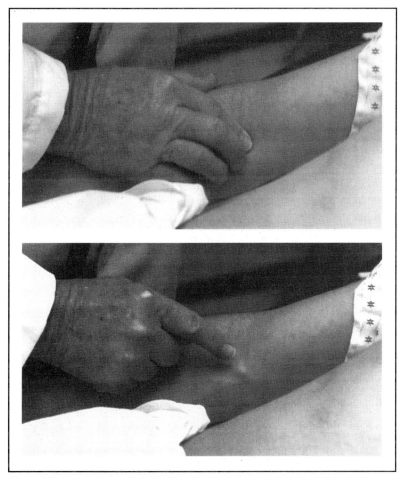

Figure 184: First Steps — Before taking the blood pressure, palpate and locate the brachial artery pulsation in the antecubital fossa. Bottom: Place the stethoscope over this area, which is more medial in location.

The auscultatory blood pressure sounds (Korotkoff Sounds) will be heard best over this area. The fact that this area is not searched for and utilized may explain why difficulty may be experienced in hearing the sounds.

Probably not well appreciated is the fact that obese patients can have their blood pressure return to normal if the excess weight is lost.

Also, spurious high blood pressure readings can be recorded in obese individuals if too small a cuff is used. Using the largest size blood pressure cuff may show a normal blood pressure (Figures 185 and 186); and for infants and children, the small size blood pressure cuff is indicated.

Also helpful in deciding when to treat the patient's hypertension is to have the patient keep a log and take his or her blood pressures several times a day, preferably by the same person. Such home recordings, with a reliable blood pressure apparatus previously checked out for accuracy by the physician, can be helpful. State in the log whether each day was a normal one, or whether there was increased stress, problems, and so forth. Review of the log at the end of several weeks usually identifies the individual who needs treatment and eliminates those with the "white coat syndrome."

After starting treatment, it is helpful to have the patient continue to keep a daily log for review by the physician; any adjustment or need for different combinations of the medical regimen quickly become evident.

Take the blood pressure in both arms. If there is a discrepancy on the second arm examined, go back to the first one to make sure it was not an insignificant normal fast drop.

• The Importance of Multiple Readings
— It is suggested that several blood pressure readings be recorded each time a patient is examined, since many will have a drop of 10 to 15 millimeters of mercury of systolic and 5 to 10 millimeters of diastolic on second or third readings taken over a period of 5 to 10 minutes.

Easy, simple application of the blood pressure cuff on the patient's arm in the supine position is shown in Figure 187. Lift the patient's right arm and hold it in place under the physician's right axilla. The physician can now easily wrap the cuff snugly to the patient's arm. Then rest the patient's arm on the examining table. Of course, in the sitting position, this is not necessary.

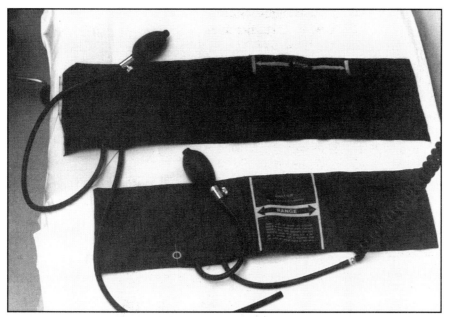

Figure 185: Large and Small — Avoid a spurious elevation of blood pressure reading using a normal sized cuff (lower) on a patient who is obese, having a very large arm. Use the larger size cuff (upper).

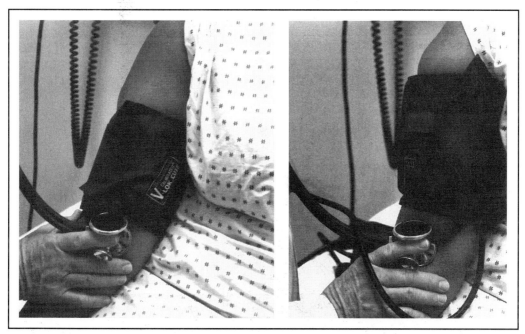

Figure 186: Use the Appropriate Size Cuff — This patient is very obese. A false elevation of blood pressure can be recorded by using the normal sized blood pressure cuff (on the left). The correct reading, which may be normal, is recorded using the larger cuff size (shown on the right).

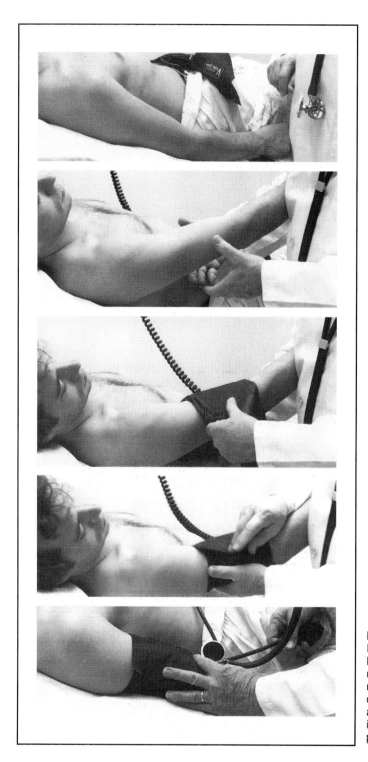

Figure 187: Easy Application —
If the patient is lying on his back,
lift his right arm and hold it in place
under your right axilla. You can
now easily wrap the blood pressure
cuff snugly to the patient's arm (3rd
and 4th panels). Bottom: The arm
is now resting while the blood
pressure is taken.

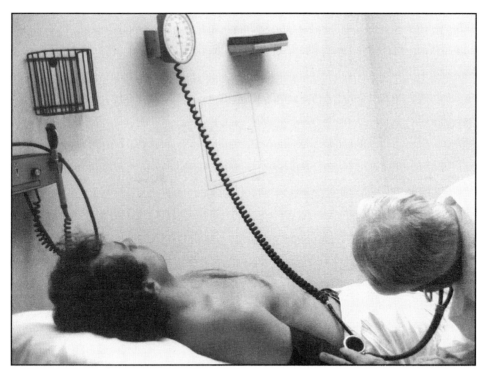

Figure 188: How Not to Take a Blood Pressure — One should not have to stand almost on one's head to see the manometer (which should be placed much lower down). This photo was actually taken in an examining room of a teaching hospital (mine)!

- *"Do it yourself" blood pressure determination* **(Figure 189). The blood pressure cuff is rolled to the proper diameter with the Velcro adhesive holding it securely. The cuff is then slipped upward over the arm to the proper place just above the antecubital fossa. The stethoscope's diaphragm can now be placed (wedged) under the cuff over the brachial arterial pulsation while you prepare for the next steps. The hand of the arm containing the cuff can be used to inflate the cuff; the other will be free to hold the stethoscope in place. The cuff can then be slipped off, keeping the same diameter and ready for use the next time.**

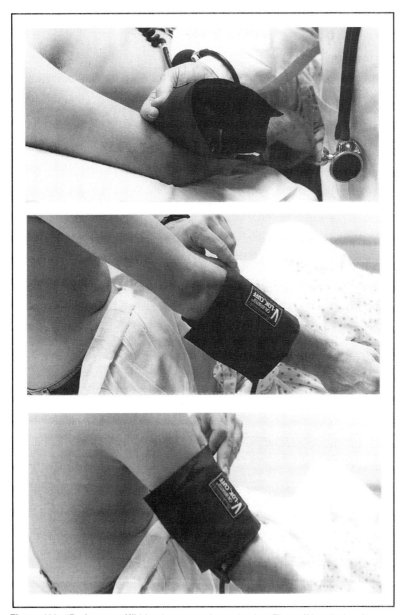

Figure 189: "Do it yourself" blood pressure determination. The cuff is rolled to the proper diameter with the velcro holding it securely (top). The cuff is then slipped into place by the patient (middle and bottom). The stethoscope can now be placed over the brachial arterial pulsation; the diaphragm chest piece is then wedged in place under the cuff. Both hands are now free to take the blood pressure. The cuff can then be slipped off keeping the same diameter and ready for use the next time.

The Stethoscope

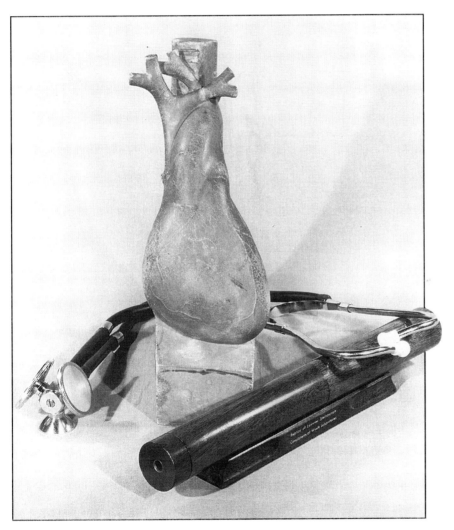

Figure 190: Replica of Rene Laennec's Original Stethoscope — The *first*, compared with a modern stethoscope.

- **How do you tell a good stethoscope from an inferior one? The answer is simple — an excellent stethoscope can pick up the faintest high frequency murmur (such as an early, blowing, aortic diastolic murmur) and the faintest low frequency sound, such as a diastolic rumble or gallop (S_3, S_4).**

If your stethoscope can't do this, discard it. You are penalizing yourself as well as the patient.

- **Use all chest pieces on each patient (Figures 191 and 192). The flat diaphragm chest piece is best for detecting a faint, early blowing aortic diastolic murmur; also for analysis of systolic clicks, ejection sounds, and most systolic murmurs. The flat diaphragm chest piece is the "work horse." As a rule, the bell is best for the detection of low frequencies, such as diastolic rumbles and faint gallop sounds.**

The diaphragm can also be used to detect low frequency sounds, although not as well as the bell piece. To pick up low frequencies with the diaphragm, just touch the skin of the chest wall very lightly; the low frequency sounds of a gallop or diastolic rumble can sometimes be readily detected. This, of course, should be done only when the bell piece is not available.

Low frequency sounds are better heard with the bell-type chest piece, again touching the skin very lightly and barely making an air seal.

- **Length of Tubing — The length of the stethoscope tubing is important. Actually, the closer one gets to the heart, and thus the shorter the tubing, the better. However, the physician must also be comfortable and a tall physician would be uncomfortable using short tubing.**

- **Eartips — From experience with postgraduate courses where one has to use the stethoscope for long periods, it has become evident to me that the eartips should be large enough to fit snugly in the ear canals, and be made of firm, smooth plastic.**

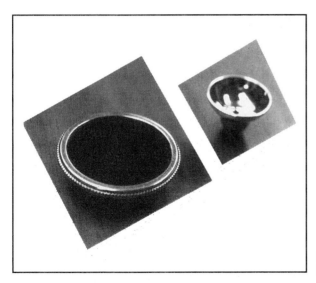

Figure 191: Two Heads — Flat diaphragm and bell chest pieces of stethoscope.

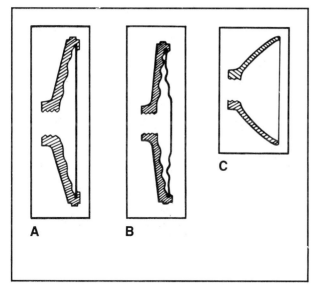

A   B   C

Figure 192: Three Heads: (A) Flat Diaphragm: "The workhorse." Excellent for all sounds and murmurs. Best for higher frequencies (such as faint diastolic murmur of aortic regurgitation). Also ideal to identify splitting of sounds, systolic clicks, and ejection sounds.
(B) Corrugated Diaphragm: Amplifying quality. Excellent for an overview of heart sounds. Especially good for low-frequency gallop sounds and murmurs.
(C) Bell: Provides excellent detection and clarity for low and medium frequency heart sounds and murmurs (such as a faint gallop or diastolic rumble).

Stethoscopes with soft rubber tips or even hard rubber tips have resulted in more discomfort and irritation for me, although some people prefer them. The small size ear tips, often of a hard material, may not fit snugly and can, in fact, cause discomfort, which I refer to as "somewhat like having a myringotomy in one's ear."

Emphasizing the importance of a good stethoscope is the following anecdote: When I first became Director of the Division of Cardiology at Georgetown, I was working on a teaching project in which we were recording heart sounds and murmurs on high fidelity tape. We produced a collection of 4½ hours of these teaching tapes and donated copies to any medical school or medical institution that requested them. We also set up a small room in our hospital with high fidelity equipment for self teaching. We named it "The Listening Post," which was printed on a heartshaped sign hanging outside the room. (The name "Listening Post" was thought appropriate since, at that time, Russia was behind the Iron Curtain allowing no visitors. The United States set up a "listening post" close to the Russian border and monitored, for intelligence purposes, communications emanating from Russia.)

Dr. Carl Wiggers (Figure 192A), one of the most eminent physiologists ever produced in the United States, somehow heard of our teaching efforts, and paid us a visit to personally observe the setup.

This nice gentleman spent several hours with us and at the end of his stay he told us this story: When he was a student in medical school he could not hear with his stethoscope the heart sounds and murmurs that the other students could. He realized that there was something wrong with his ability to hear. This problem continued in his postgraduate training and he accepted the fact that this was a defect that he would have to put up with.

He then went into the field of physiology, in which he excelled. He subsequently worked at the Rockefeller Institute in New York City. Returning to his home one evening and crossing one of the major New York bridges in heavy traffic, the headlights of his automobile failed. In the midst of this predicament, he sought to find the problem with the lights, which had an acetylene source (Figure 192B). He discovered that there was a break in the "Y" tube leading from the acetylene source to the two headlights. Wondering how he could fix it, he remembered that his old stethoscope was in a bag in his car. Sure enough, his stethoscope had a metal "Y" piece with which he was able to replace the broken part of his automobile light system. It worked!

However, when he got home and drove into his garage, he noticed there was only one light illuminated, not two! The next morning he secured the correct replacement part; he took his stethoscope "Y" piece to his laboratory for close examination.

Yes, you guessed it! One bore of the "Y" piece had never been opened. Dr. Wiggers therefore went through medical school and postgraduate training "on one ear."

I said to him as he was leaving, "Dr. Wiggers, it was fortunate for science that this happened. Otherwise you might have become a cardiologist."

- **Reverse Listening — I recently learned that Dr. William S. Nevin of Tucson, Arizona, helps his hard of hearing patients by putting his stethoscope in their ears and speaking into the chest piece. The patient's hearing is thereby enhanced. I have tried this and it does amplify one's voice to the patient. Thanks, Dr. Nevin, for that cardiac pearl.**

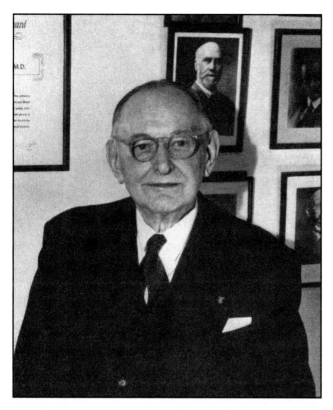

- **If you listen with only one ear, you might become a renowned physiologist.**

Figure 192A: Dr. Carl Wiggers

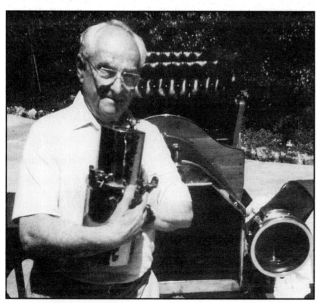

Figure 192B: Acetylene Source, as described by Dr. Carl Wiggers, for headlights of his automobile.
Courtesy Dr. Allen Johnson, Scripps Clinic, La Jolla, California

Arterial and Venous Pulses

- **The Significance of a Paradoxical Pulse** — The term "paradoxical pulse" is really a misnomer because when it is clinically apparent, it is really only an exaggeration of the normal pulse. The decrease in amplitude of the pulse coincident with inspiration may be of help in diagnosing constrictive pericarditis. Paradoxical pulse also is an important sign of pericardial tamponade, and may be a sign of restrictive cardiomyopathy, or chronic pulmonary disease such as emphysema or asthma.

- **Aneurysm** — How to differentiate between an aneurysm and a buckled subclavian or carotid artery.

    Some elderly patients are prone to elongation and tortuosity of the aorta, which in turn may result in buckling of the carotid and/or subclavian arteries in the neck. Most often, these are easily seen and palpated, but sometimes a buckled carotid is erroneously interpreted as an aneurysm. To distinguish between the two one can usually outline the caliber and course of the buckled vessel by simple palpation, using two fingers such as the thumb and index on each side outlining it, noting that coincident with systole there is an outward thrust of the vessel. A buckled artery causes no symptoms and is benign.

- **Significance of a bisferiens pulse.**

    A double systolic impulse in the radial, brachial, carotid or femoral arterial pulse is called a bisferiens pulse. When this is present, think of three possibilities: 1. A combination of aortic stenosis plus aortic regurgitation; 2. More severe aortic regurgitation; 3. Hypertrophic cardiomyopathy.

- **Palpation of Arterial Pulses** — Valuable information concerning abnormalities of arterial pulsation await us if we look for these pulses... and know what we are looking for. Figures 193, 194 and 195 identify the sites of various arterial pulsations.

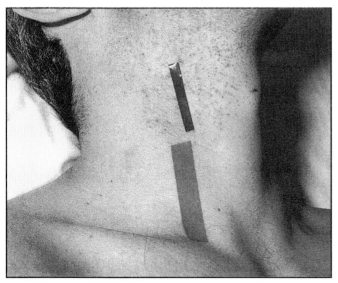

Figure 193: Pulses — The carotid arterial pulse is medial to the mid-line of the neck. The jugular venous pulse (larger marker) is lateral. It is helpful to see both pulsations simultaneously. If the jugular pulse precedes the carotid, this is an A-wave; if they are occurring at the same times, this is a V-wave of the jugular pulse.

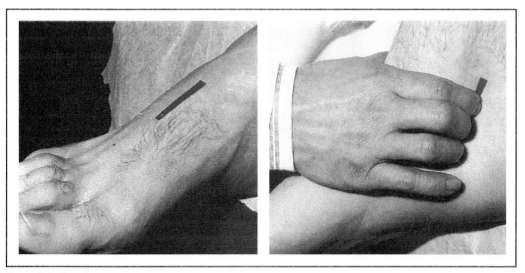

Figure 194: More Pulses — Sites of palpation of the dorsalis pedis and posterior tibial arterial pulsations.

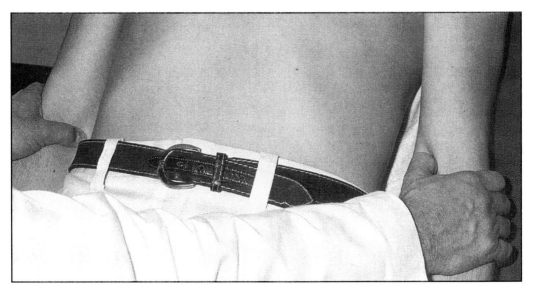

Figure 195: Simultaneous Palpation — Simultaneous palpation of the brachial arterial pulsations should be done to note any inequality.

Jugular Venous Pulse

- **The best way to detect the specific waves of the jugular venous pulse in the neck is to be able to *see* both the venous pulsation and the carotid arterial pulsation in the same localized area. If this can be done, remember that the venous pulsation is lateral and the arterial is medial. (Figure 193)**

If we detect a pulsation of the jugular vein just before that of the carotid artery, then this has to be an A-wave. Sometimes this cannot be seen, but it is worth the time to concentrate using only one sense, the visual. If it is not possible to visualize this pulsation, then the carotid arterial pulsation (on the same side or opposite side) can be felt with the thumb or finger, noting that the venous impulse preceded the arterial; this would represent an A-wave.

When both the arterial and venous waves occur simultaneously, this would be a V-wave or CV-wave.

Of course, timing can be accomplished by palpating the carotid artery pulsation, or listening to the first heart sound, and correlating it with the jugular pulse.

- **There are only a few conditions that cause a "giant" A-wave in the jugular venous pulse:**

1. Obstruction between the right atrium and the right ventricle occuring with tricuspid stenosis or atresia, or right atrial myxoma, can cause a prominent A-wave with atrial systole.

2. Increased pressure in the right ventricle, as may occur from severe obstruction of the pulmonary outflow tract with pulmonic stenosis, will result in a significant A-wave on atrial contraction.

3. Pulmonary hypertension ("Eisenmenger syndrome" — pulmonary hypertension, with atrial defect, ventricular defect, and patent ductus arteriosus) can cause pressure to be reflected back to the right ventricle, which produces an A-wave with atrial systole.

4. Primary pulmonary hypertension (unknown etiology).

5. Recurrent pulmonary emboli can produce a prominent A-wave of the jugular venous pulse.

The First Heart Sound

As a rule, the first heart sound is normal in intensity. The length of the P-R interval on the electrocardiogram is related to the intensity of the first heart sound. If there is a short P-R interval, the first heart sound is accentuated (eg, 0.14 or 0.15 seconds). If the P-R interval is prolonged, the first sound is faint (eg, 0.19-0.22 seconds or longer) (Figures 196 and 197).

When one hears a loud first heart sound in a patient whose heart rate is normal, think of two possibilities: A short P-R interval on the electrocardiogram and mitral stenosis. In fact, the loud first sound of a short P-R can be misdiagnosed as that of mitral stenosis; if a normal physiological third sound is also present, it too can be misinterpreted as an opening snap (Figure 197).

Splitting of Heart Sounds: Splitting of the first sound is due to closure of the mitral valve followed by tricuspid valve closure. The second sound split is due to aortic valve closure followed by tricuspid valve closure.

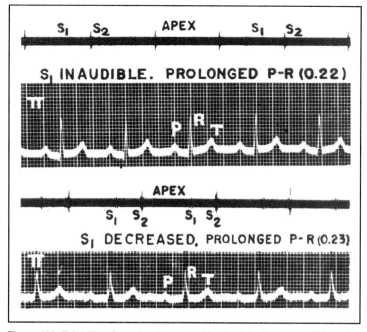

Figure 196: Faint First Sound — If searched for, the faint first sound (S_1) can be readily detected with one's stethoscope.

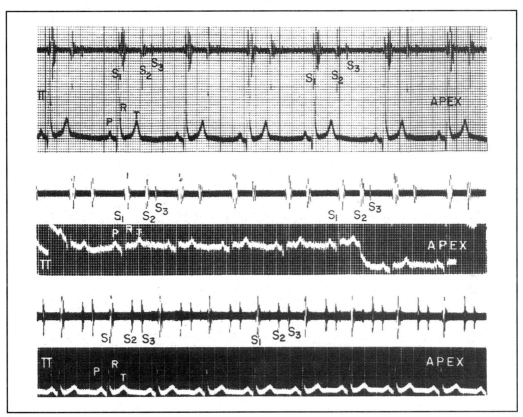

Figure 197: The loud first sound (S₁) in each patient is due to a short P-R interval. The normal third sound usually occurs later in timing after the second sound than the opening snap of mitral stenosis. There is no evidence of heart disease in the above patients. Also, note the normal "waxing and waning" of the third sound, which is not a feature of the opening snap.

Normally, left sided events of the heart occur before the right; therefore the mitral valve closure component occurs before the tricuspid valve closure component of the first heart sound and the aortic valve closure before the pulmonic valve closure of the second heart sound.

- **The mitral component is generally louder than the tricuspid component of the first heart sound, so when the tricuspid component is louder, two conditions should immediately come to mind: Ebstein's anomaly and atrial septal defect.**

A question frequently asked: "I hear splitting of the first sound; why is this?" Splitting of the first sound usually is a normal occurrence in a healthy heart. We find it if we look for it. However, when it is more widely split than usual it may still be normal, but also can be a clue to an abnormality.

- **Wide Splitting** — **Wide splitting of the first heart sound can occur with complete left bundle branch block, complete right bundle branch block, Ebstein's anomaly, and at times with premature ventricular beats.**

Splitting of the first sound can be confused with an atrial sound (S_4) plus a first sound, or a first sound plus an ejection sound. How to tell the difference?

- **Press firmly with the diaphragm of your stethoscope against the skin of the chest wall at the lower left sternal border and/or apex.**

The S_4 will disappear. The two components of the split first sound are not eliminated with pressure; they sound alike and at the aortic area only *one* component of the split S_1 is heard. The aortic ejection sound is also usually well heard at the apex as well as over the aortic area; pressure with the stethoscope does not eliminate it and it is not affected by respiration. The pulmonic ejection sound is usually not heard at the apex and it may decrease in intensity coincident with inspiration.

Second Heart Sound

The importance of careful analysis of splitting of heart sounds, particularly that of the second heart sound, is well established and is on a firm physiologic basis. Accurate clinical diagnosis of certain types of heart disease (such as atrial septal defect) cannot be made without paying detailed attention to splitting of heart sounds. To be noted are the intensity (loudness) and the degree of splitting of the second sound, which varies from a single or closely split sound to that of a wide split. Also to be noted is the effect of inspiration and expiration on the splitting of the second sound.

- **Splitting of the *second heart sound* is usually best appreciated over the pulmonic area or the third left sternal border. Most normal hearts have a split sound over these areas. With expiration, the splitting becomes closer or may even become single, and coincident with inspiration there is an increase in the degree of splitting.**

With inspiration, venous return of blood to the right side of the heart is increased; pulmonic valve closure (P_2) is thereby delayed, because the right ventricle requires a little more time to pump this normally increased volume of blood to the lungs.

At the same time, with inspiration there is a slight, earlier closure of the aortic valve (A_2), which is another factor contributing to the wider splitting of the second heart sound (Figure 198). However, the most striking change on inspiration is the normal delay in closure of the pulmonic valve.

- **When some patients are lying in the supine position, their second heart sound is distinctly split, thereby raising the possibility of atrial septal defect or bundle branch block. If on sitting or standing the sound becomes single or closely split, it tells you that the heart is normal.**

This is more common in children, but also can occur in adults, especially athletes. We found this frequently in a number of National Football League players.

It is important to select the best spot over the pulmonic area or left sternal border where the two components of the second heart sound can be readily and clearly heard. The flat diaphragm of the stethoscope is usually the best chest piece to detect splitting of heart sounds.

The patient's respiration should be normal and quiet, the mouth slightly opened. It is important that the patient not force deep respirations. A helpful technique is to have the patient follow your free hand and to inspire when the hand moves upward, and exhale when it moves downward.

The splitting of the second heart sound has a significant relationship to various pathologic cardiac conditions. As might be expected, those disorders that delay contraction of the right side of the heart also result in delayed closure of the pulmonary valve. Therefore, even in expiration an increased degree of splitting might be present, and with inspiration there is an additional widening of the components of the second heart sound.

Complete right bundle branch block is a good illustration of this: Since there is an electrical delay of activation of the right side of the heart, the left ventricle contracts on schedule while there is some delay in right ventricular contraction. Therefore, with expiration there is a wider than normal splitting of the second heart sound, and with inspiration there is an additional increase in the normal degree of splitting.

Wider splitting of the second heart sound may also be heard in patients with right ventricular outflow obstruction. This occurs, for example, in patients with valvular or subvalvular pulmonic stenosis (Figure 199). Obstruction of outflow from the right ventricle results. Thus, pulmonic valve closure is delayed, because it takes longer for the right ventricle to empty its contents.

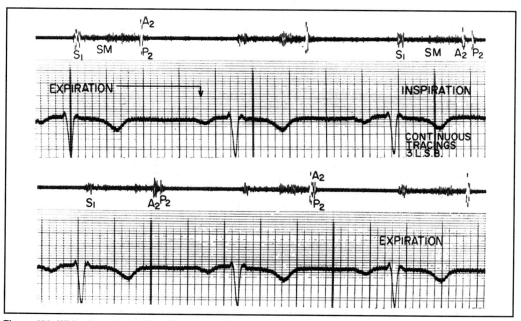

Figure 198: Widening of the Split — These tracings show normal increase in splitting of the second heart sound on inspiration. This splitting is easily detected with the flat diaphragm of the stethoscope. Also, note holosystolic murmur (SM).

- **The wider the degree of splitting in pulmonic stenosis, the more severe the obstruction.**

As the severity of stenosis increases, the second heart sound becomes prolonged and progressively fainter. Also, with increases in the degree of stenosis, the harsh "diamond-shaped" or "kite-shaped" murmur of pulmonic stenosis becomes more prolonged, extending to, or even subsequently masking, the aortic valve closure sound so that one hears only the faint, delayed pulmonic valve closure (Figure 199).

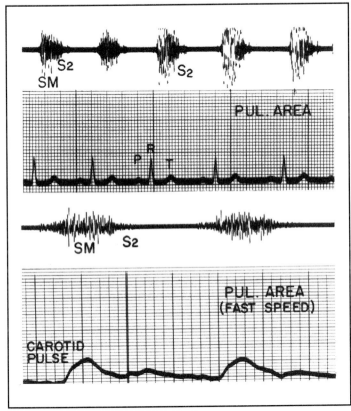

Figure 199: Fainter Second Sound — This patient has significant valvular pulmonic stenosis. The second sound (S₂) is delayed and faint.

Atrial Septal Defect

- **A real cardiac pearl and an auscultatory finding that has withstood the test of time is the wide splitting of the second heart sound present with atrial septal defect (Figure 200).**

In fact, when one hears wider splitting of the second heart sound over the pulmonic area or third left sternal border, and this does not become single or very closely split with expiration, then the possibility of atrial septal defect must be considered, particularly if a pulmonic systolic murmur is also present. I have observed many patients whose very first bedside clue to atrial septal defect was the presence of a wider split of the second heart sound.

- **In the presence of atrial septal defect, the second heart sound can simulate that of complete right bundle branch block; however, one major difference is that patients with right bundle branch block often have no murmur over the pulmonic area as do patients with atrial septal defect.**

It is rare that a grade 2 or grade 3 systolic murmur is not heard in early or mid portions of systole in patients with atrial septal defect (Figure 200).

In addition, with complete right bundle branch block, the second heart sound generally has more movement than the so-called "fixed" splitting of atrial septal defect. This fixed splitting of the second heart sound has been emphasized by Dr. Aubrey Leatham and his colleagues in London. Although the splitting is wide and is still heard as split with expiration, there may be very slight widening of the split coinciding with inspiration; this is detectable on auscultation in about one third of patients with proven atrial septal defect. When the patient sits up or stands, the wide, fixed splitting remains.

This wide splitting is due to the increased volume of blood shunted to the right side of the heart with the more common (ostium secundum) type of atrial septal defect. It also may occur with ostium primum defect.

- **Often the only clue to an ostium primum defect is left axis deviation on the electrocardiogram.**

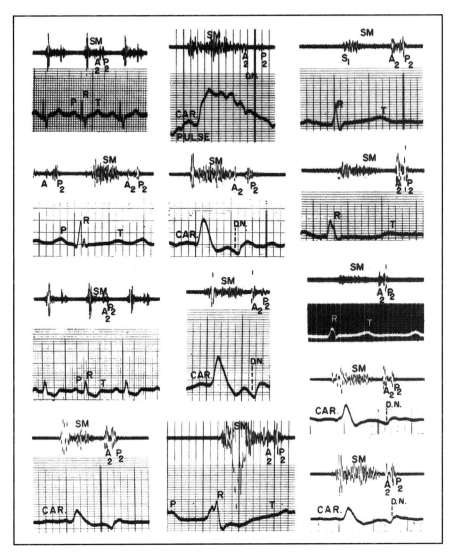

Figure 200: Thirteen patients with atrial septal defect (ostium secundum type). The second sound (A_2, P_2) did not become single or closely split with expiration. Note systolic murmur (SM) of each patient. The absence of a systolic murmur practically rules out the diagnosis of atrial septal defect.

Also, with the larger shunts at the atrial level, a "flow" rumbling murmur may be heard along the lower left sternal border; this is the result of the increased flow of blood shunted from the left atrium to the right side of the heart, producing a more turbulent flow across the tricuspid valve.

Some patients, particularly children with an innocent murmur heard over the right ventricular outflow tract, may have a murmur very similar to that associated with atrial septal defect. Characteristically, innocent murmurs are short in duration, occurring in early to mid portions of systole. They are frequently heard over the pulmonic area or third left sternal border, just as murmurs of atrial septal defects are heard.

Of course, occasionally an innocent pulmonic systolic murmur can be present in a patient having right bundle branch block. However, the total cardiovascular evaluation can make the correct diagnosis. For instance, the chest x-ray will show the atrial defect with an enlarged pulmonary artery segment, plus increased vascular markings. Also the innocent murmur will often be heard in more than one area: over the aortic area, left sternal border, apex, precordium, rather than localized over the third left sternal border or pulmonic area.

At times there may be noticeable splitting of the second heart sound with expiration, with the split becoming even wider with inspiration. A grade 2 or 3 early to mid systolic murmur is heard over the third left sternal border and/or over the pulmonic area. Is this atrial septal defect or an innocent systolic murmur?

- **A simple maneuver is to have the patient sit or stand up; if the second sound then becomes single, or very closely split on expiration, this is most likely a normal variant, and not the wide splitting of atrial septal defect. However, "never say never"...Occasionally, a small atrial septal defect can have a single or closely split S_2 with expiration.**

- **Also remember that the *absence* of a systolic murmur (even faint) heard over the pulmonic area or left sternal border practically eliminates the diagnosis of atrial septal defect.**

If the sound becomes single when the patient is sitting, atrial septal defect would be an unlikely diagnosis. Athletes such as professional football players may have similar findings, as described with the children (See discussion on innocent murmurs). All aspects of the total cardiovascular picture should be put together, using the "five-finger approach," which includes a carefully detailed history, physical examination, electrocardiogram, chest x-ray, and laboratory tests. Then one can generally easily determine whether the patient has an innocent murmur.

For example, a patient with atrial septal defect would have wide, fixed splitting of the second heart sound and a systolic murmur of grade 2 or 3. There would be electrocardiographic changes, particularly noted in V_1, such as right ventricular conduction delay, indicated by an RSR_1. Or the patient would have incomplete right bundle branch block, complete right bundle branch block, or right ventricular hypertrophy. The x-ray would show an enlarged pulmonary artery segment with increased vascular markings, and the echocardiogram might show findings consistent with atrial septal defect. The echocardiogram and cardiac catheterization could, of course, document this.

- **To diagnose an Innocent Murmur: If the second sound does not become single or closely split with expiration, it might do so with the patient sitting upright or standing. The patient's history and auscultatory findings would be negative except for the systolic murmur; the electrocardiogram and x-ray would be normal.**

Further evidence of an innocent murmur is the finding of a short vibratory murmur (often with a buzzing quality — so-called Still's murmur), which may be an immediate indication of innocence. In addition, the absence of an ejection sound with the innocent murmur is further evidence, but suggests the possibility of milder degrees of pulmonic stenosis; at times, the ejection sound can be heard in patients with atrial septal defect, although it is much more common with congenital valvular pulmonic stenosis.

After surgical closure of atrial septal defects, splitting of the second sound is sometimes normalized (Figure 201); in others the splitting narrows, but never totally normalizes.

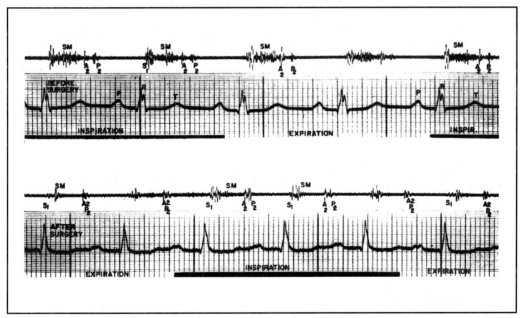

Figure 201: Atrial Septal Defect — Note splitting of second sound (A_2, P_2) is "fixed" before surgical correction (top panel) and becomes more normal with expiration after surgery (bottom panel).

- **Wide splitting of the second heart sound also can be found in patients with anomalous venous return (Figure 202). This defect is often associated with atrial septal defect but, uncommonly, it does occur alone; in such cases the second heart sound is more likely to have more movement of the split with respiration than that of the typically "fixed splitting" of atrial septal defect.**

Just as delay of the pulmonic component with inspiration results in wider splitting, earlier closure of the aortic component can produce wider splitting of the second heart sound. An example of this is mitral regurgitation of more advanced degrees in which the more significant leaks of the incompetent mitral valve result in earlier emptying of the contents of the left ventricle, thereby producing an early closure of the aortic valve (Figure 203).

- **Wider splitting can also occur in patients with large ventricular septal defects; the mechanism is similar to that of mitral regurgitation.**

In this instance, the aortic closure is earlier due to more rapid emptying of left ventricular blood caused by the "run-off" through the ventricular septal defect; this is concomitant with the ejection of blood to the aorta. Wide splitting of the second heart sound may also occur with idiopathic dilatation of the pulmonary artery and the straight back syndrome.

- **With paradoxical splitting of the second heart sound, the reverse of normal splitting takes place. Instead of the degree of splitting increasing with inspiration, the splitting is wider with expiration and more closely split or single with inspiration.**

For example, complete left bundle branch block (Figure 204) is associated with delayed electrical conduction to the left side of the heart, which thereby delays left ventricular contraction.

While aortic valve closure normally precedes pulmonic valve closure, in patients with left bundle branch block the order may be reversed. With expiration, therefore, P_2 may occur before A_2, with inspiration P_2 moves toward it, resulting in close splitting, or a single second sound; with expiration the splitting is wider again.

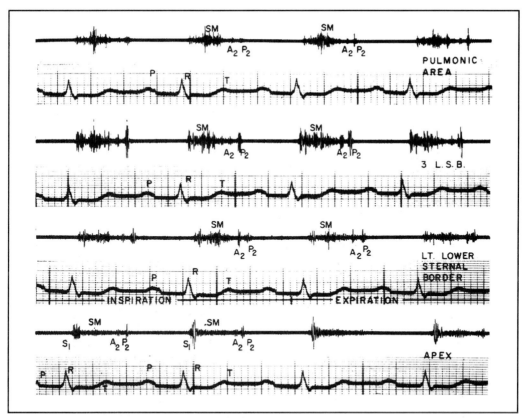

Figure 202: Anomalous Pulmonary Venous Drainage — Note systolic murmur (SM) and persistent wide split of the second sound (A₂, P₂) with both inspiration and expiration.

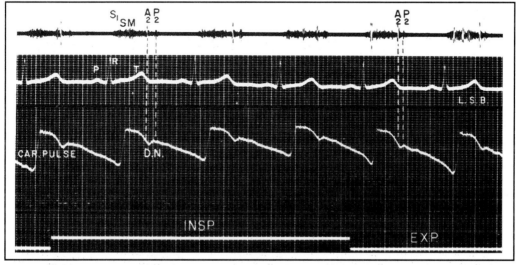

Figure 203: Mitral Insufficiency — The splitting of the second sound (A₂, P₂) is wide with both inspiration and expiration.

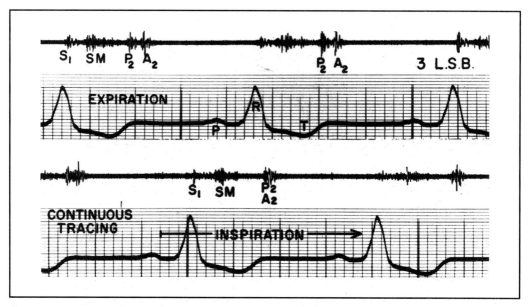

Figure 204: Left Bundle Branch Block — Note the pulmonic valve component (P$_2$) of the second sound occurs before the delayed aortic component (A$_2$). The second sound becomes closely split with inspiration and wider on expiration.

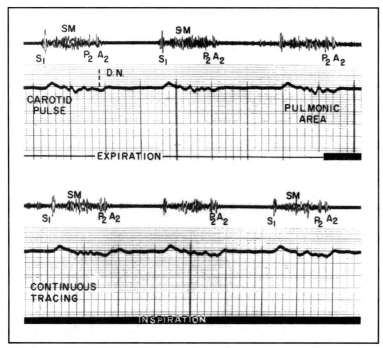

Figure 205: Paradoxical Splitting of Aortic Stenosis — The normal splitting of the second sound (A$_2$, P$_2$) is *reversed:* Aortic valve closure (A$_2$) occurs *after* the pulmonic valve closure (P$_2$). Note the closer split with inspiration.

- **Paradoxical splitting of S_2 can occur with aortic outflow obstruction (Figure 205). It is more likely to occur with hypertrophic cardiomyopathy than valvular aortic stenosis.**

Most physicians report difficulty in detecting the various degrees of splitting. It is merely a matter of practicing concentration on the second heart sound and hearing successive degrees of synchrony of sounds. Any physician can become expert in the bedside detection of the spectrum of splitting of sounds. This can be simulated by striking two knuckles or fingertips on a hard surface (Figure 206); one can easily vary the degree of synchrony. Striking only one knuckle produces a single sound. Striking both knuckles not quite simultaneously imitates a close split, and a wide split is simulated by delaying the second knuckle before striking it. The tips of the fingers on one hand can also be used in place of the knuckles as just described.

It is also possible, using this technique, to simulate the first sound, second sound, opening snap — all in proper sequence. Many physicians have been able to apply what they have learned from this technique to the accurate auscultation of actual patients.

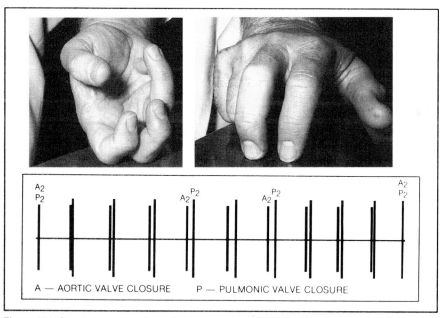

Figure 206: Simulation of heart sounds by striking knuckles or fingertips on a hard surface.

- **Atrial Septal Defect (Figures 207, 208 and 209) vs Pulmonic Stenosis (Figure 210)**

Ostium secundum septal defect and a mild congenital pulmonic valve stenosis can have both a similar murmur and a wider split of the second sound that does not become single on expiration. How to tell the difference?

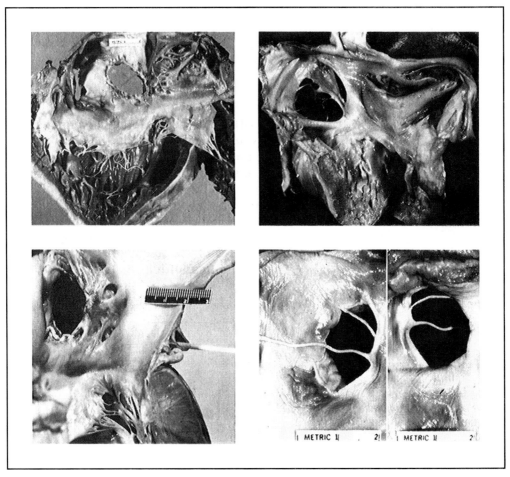

Figure 207: Atrial Septal Defect — Four patients with atrial septal defect — ostium secundum type. Defect viewed from both left and right atrium (lower right).

- **Presence of a pulmonic systolic ejection sound immediately indicates pulmonic stenosis. This ejection sound may decrease in intensity or disappear on inspiration.**

- **Variation in splitting — The wide, so-called "fixed splitting," of the second heart sound in patients with atrial septal defect is not "fixed" in approximately 25% of patients, who may have some degree of increase in widening coincident with inspiration. The increase may be slight, but with careful auscultation it can be detected.**

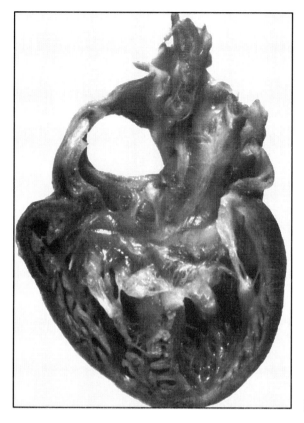

Figure 208: Large atrial septal defect.

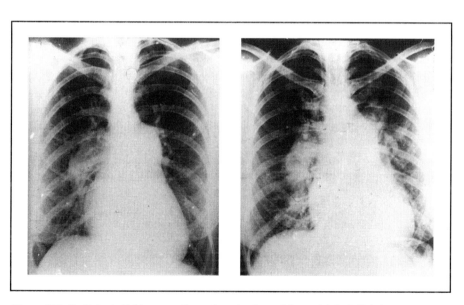

Figure 209: Radiologic Evidence — Two patients having atrial septal defect. Note large pulmonary arteries and increased vascular markings.

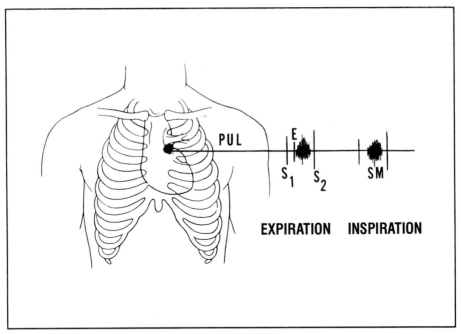

Figure 210: Valvular Pulmonic Stenosis — The ejection sound (E) disappears (or becomes fainter) with inspiration. SM = systolic murmur. AO = aortic area. Pul = pulmonic area.

It is interesting that on routine examination of a large number of professional football players, the majority had wider split of the second heart sound with inspiration. A grade 1 to 3 early to mid-systolic innocent murmur was also heard. The splitting of the second sound did not become single or closely split with expiration. However, on sitting and/or standing the splitting did become single or closely split, as normally occurs. Therefore, atrial defect was not a consideration (Figure 211).

Let's consider another situation. A 17-year-old boy has a grade 2 to 3 early to mid-systolic murmur best heard over the pulmonic area. The second sound is more widely split with inspiration than usual and does not become single or closely split with expiration (Figure 212). Is this atrial septal defect? Is there anything else we can do at the bedside to help differentiate between atrial septal defect and a normal variant of splitting of the second heart sound? Yes. Have the patient sit and/or stand up. The second sound may now become single or closely split on expiration. This indicates a variant of normal splitting of the second sound plus an innocent systolic murmur. In such patients the EKG and chest x-ray will also be normal.

- **Contrary to common belief, the second sound can, on expiration, become single or closely split in the presence of uncomplicated ostium secundum atrial septal defect. This is unusual, however. If this occurs, the defect is generally small in size.**

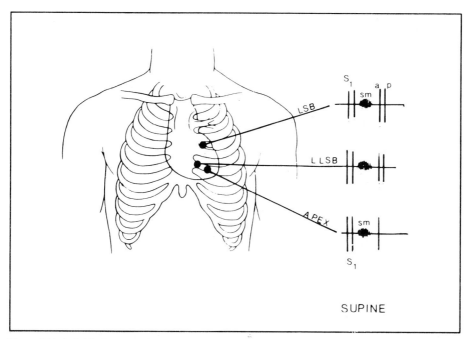

Figure 211: Atrial Defect? No — The patient is an all-Pro NFL football player lying supine. Note wide split of first sound (S_1), innocent systolic murmur (sm), and wide split of S_2 (a-p) which did not become single on expiration. However, it did become single on expiration in the sitting position.

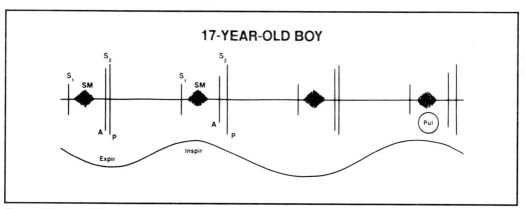

Figure 212: Normal Heart — The second heart sound (A-P) is more widely split than usual. There is an innocent pulmonic systolic murmur (SM).

- **Differentiating the Ostium Primum Type** — The findings with the ostium primum type of atrial septal defect can be about the same as with the most common type, the ostium secundum. However, in some patients with the primum type a holosystolic murmur of mitral regurgitation can also be present.

The presence of left axis deviation on the electrocardiogram should be an immediate clue to change the diagnosis of secundum defect to that of primum defect (Figures 213 and 214).

- **Unless lead V₁ of the ECG shows RSR₁, right ventricular conduction delay, right bundle branch block, or right ventricular hypertrophy, be cautious in making the diagnosis of atrial septal defect. The great majority of patients with atrial septal defect will have one of these findings (Figure 213).**

- **Absence of a Systolic Murmur — The *absence* of a systolic murmur practically rules out the diagnosis of uncomplicated ostium secundum atrial septal defect.**

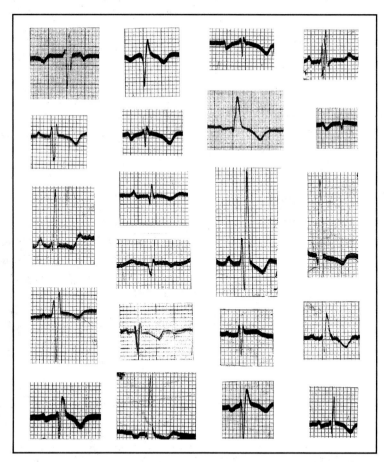

Figure 213: Twenty-one Examples — Lead V₁ of 21 patients with atrial septal defect. One of these patterns is present in approximately 90% of patients with ASD.

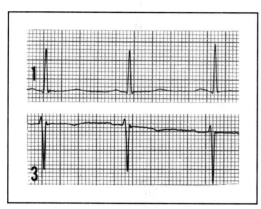

Figure 214: Differentiating Primum From Secundum
— Tracing shows left axis deviation. Ostium primum
atrial septal defect can simulate the most common type,
ostium secundum. However, if left axis deviation is
present on the electrocardiogram, suspect ostium
primum.

Causes of a Loud
Second Heart Sound

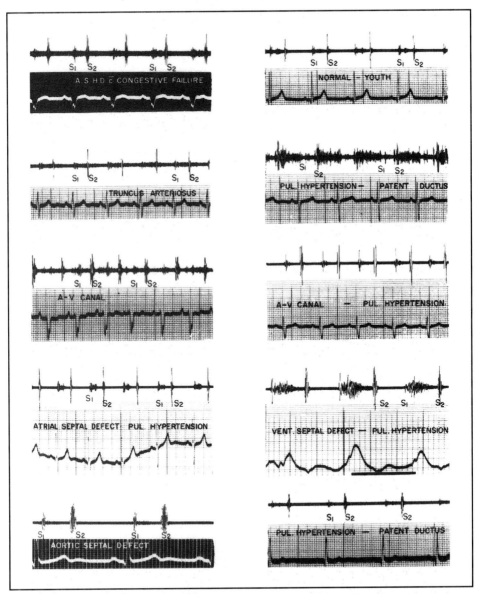

Figure 215: Ten Patients — Various causes of an accentuated second sound (S_2) of the pulmonic valve closure.

The pulmonic valve closure becomes accentuated (Figure 215) with heart failure. As already discussed, the closure of P_2 correlates with the additional time needed to empty the blood from the right ventricle that has been received with inspiration. However, in the presence of severe right ventricular failure, this respiratory variation in splitting may no longer occur; the right ventricle has already failed and cannot readily accommodate the extra blood coming into the right ventricle with inspiration. In this circumstance, there may be little or no change in the time of closure of the pulmonic valve. Splitting of S_2 remains wide in both expiration and inspiration.

Particularly with more advanced degrees of cardiac decompensation, one may detect little or no change in the splitting of the second heart sound with respiration as would otherwise occur with right or left bundle branch block (Figure 216).

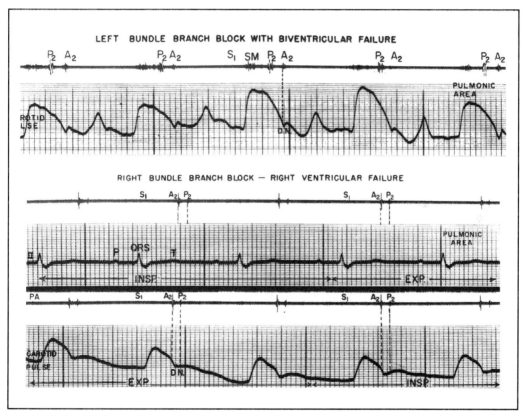

Figure 216: Heart Failure — Two patients with advanced heart failure. Top photo shows a patient with LBBB and biventricular failure. Bottom shows RBBB and right ventricular failure. The usual respiratory change of splitting of the second heart sound is not present. Note splitting of S_2 is wide in both expiration and inspiration.

The Second Heart Sound: Pulmonary Hypertension

- **As a rule, with pulmonary hypertension of a significant degree, the pulmonic component of the second sound becomes greatly accentuated and splitting usually becomes closer (Figures 215, 217, and 218). Pulmonary hypertension of this kind may occur with ventricular septal defect, atrial septal defect, patent ductus arteriosus, primary pulmonary hypertension, or recurrent pulmonary emboli.**

The second heart sound becomes quite loud and easily palpable. This is because of the accentuated pulmonary valve component. In addition, an ejection sound frequently may be heard. Particularly with the ventricular Eisenmenger defect, the second sound is often described as single. With inspiration, however, patients with pulmonary hypertension generally show a slight widening of the components of the second heart sound, which can be detected by the ear.

If pulmonary hypertension is associated with an atrial septal defect, more distinct splitting of the second heart sound generally is heard and is one clinical clue to atrial defect (Figure 218). This is distinguished from other causes of the Eisenmenger syndrome, such as ventricular septal defect.

In the case of patent ductus with associated pulmonary hypertension, the typically continuous "machinery" murmur enveloping the second heart sound is replaced by either a murmur in systole alone or a systolic murmur with a diastolic component not resembling the previous continuous murmur of ductus. I recall one patient who had no significant murmur but instead had a pulmonic ejection sound and a loud pulmonary valve closure (P_2).

Associated pulmonary valve insufficiency may develop, and in addition to a systolic murmur, one may also hear an early blowing decrescendo murmur that simulates the murmur of aortic insufficiency.

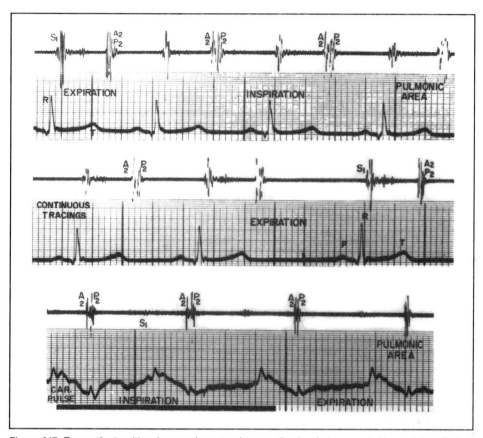

Figure 217: Two patients with pulmonary hypertension complicating their congenital heart defect. Both have closely split accentuated second sounds (A$_2$, P$_2$) that become wider with inspiration.

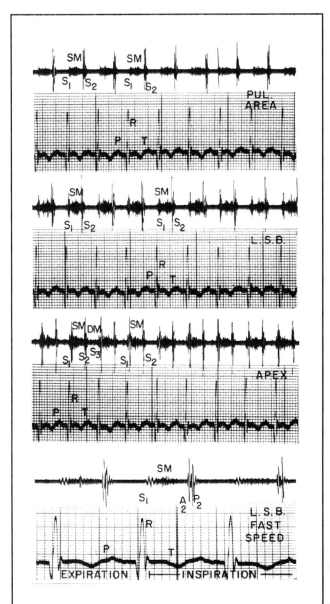

Figure 218: Atrial Septal Defect and Pulmonary Hypertension — The second sound (S$_2$) is loud and very closely split (A$_2$, P$_2$ in lower tracing). Note slight increase in the degree of splitting coincident with inspiration.

Single Second Heart Sound

A single second sound heard both in inspiration and expiration is abnormal. It is an expected finding in a cyanotic patient with classic Tetralogy of Fallot (large ventricular septal defect, severe pulmonic stenosis, and a systolic murmur). The aortic component represents the single component; P_2 may be so faint due to low pressure on the pulmonary circuit that it cannot be detected with the stethoscope over the precordium (although it may be recorded by an intracardiac phonocardiogram) (Figures 219 and 220).

Truncus arteriosus at times has a second heart sound described as single. However, careful auscultation often enables one to hear duration of the second heart sound, and indeed, in some patients one can detect an additional sound rather than only a single component.

A patient with ventricular septal defect with severe pulmonary hypertension (Eisenmenger) may be described as having a single second sound. However, I find that with careful listening, very close splitting, particularly with inspiration, may be noted in these patients.

There may be a single second heart sound, as already discussed, in more severe forms of pulmonic stenosis, with the aortic valve closure masked by a prolonged systolic murmur. Similarly, in some patients with mitral regurgitation and septal defect, a loud holosystolic murmur may obscure the aortic valve closure, which might have an earlier closure anyway in these patients. In a few patients with severe aortic valvular stenosis, aortic closure may be very faint or even absent.

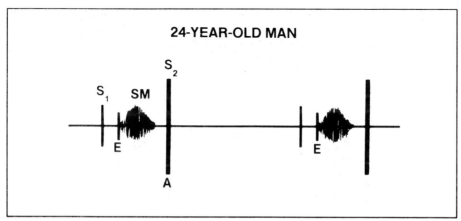

Figure 219: Classic Tetralogy of Fallot characterized by a single second sound (A$_2$), ejection sound (E), and a midsystolic murmur (SM).

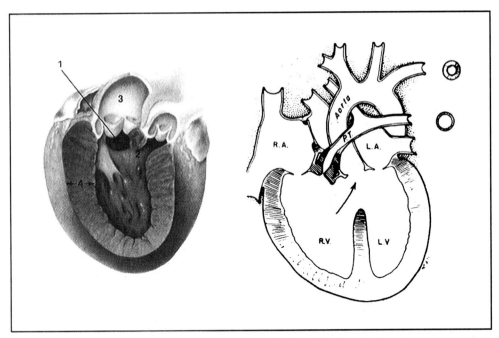

Figure 220: Tetralogy of Fallot — Note: (1) ventricular septal defect; (2) pulmonic stenosis (infundibular); (3) overriding of aorta; (4) right ventricular hypertrophy. On the diagram, notice right to left shunt and severe pulmonary stenosis. P.T. = pulmonary trunk.

- At times, the physician may not hear one component of the second heart sound because he has not listened carefully over the precordium to find the best area to hear the splitting. Difficulty may arise because of a patient's obesity or chest configuration. However, careful auscultation will generally reveal that there are two components to the second heart sound.

Pericarditis

- **Pericardial Friction Rub: There are two or three components of a true friction rub; if only a scratchy systolic murmur is heard, don't call it pericarditis (Figures 221, 222, and 223).**

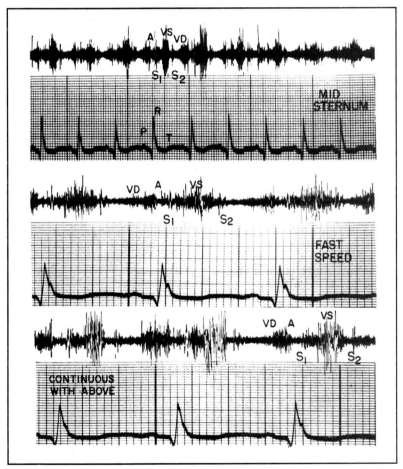

Figure 221: Three Component Friction Rub — A = Atrial systolic component. VS = Ventricular systolic component. VD = Ventricular diastolic component. Note that the friction rub becomes louder with inspiration (lower tracing).

The systolic component is related to ventricular systole (VS). The ventricular diastolic component (VD) occurs at the time of rapid filling of the ventricles and the presystolic atrial systolic component (AS) occurs before the first heart sound. If regular sinus rhythm is present, usually the three components are heard. However, if atrial fibrillation is present, there are only two components, the ventricular systolic and ventricular diastolic — since, in the presence of atrial fibrillation, there is no atrial systolic contraction, this component of the friction rub is absent.

The friction rub generally increases in intensity with inspiration.

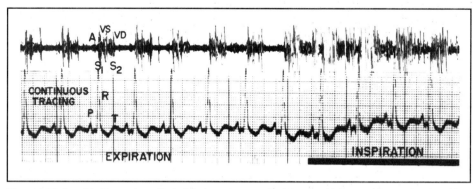

Figure 222: Another Example — Typical three component friction rub, which generally gets louder with inspiration. A = Atrial systolic component. VS = Ventricular systolic component. VD = Ventricular diastolic component.

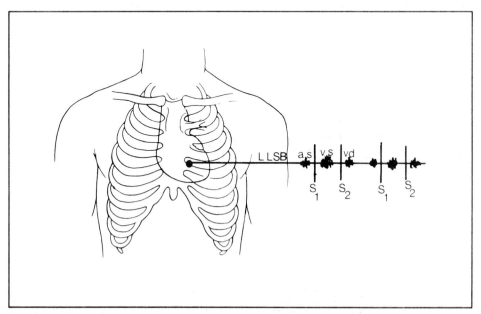

Figure 223: Sketching the Rub — A three component pericardial friction rub in a man who has an acute myocardial infarction. The three components are: 1. Atrial systolic (as). 2. Ventricular systolic (vs). 3. Ventricular diastolic (vd). LLSB = Lower left sternal border.

- **A friction rub is usually best heard over the third or fourth left sternal border using the diaphragm chest piece of the stethoscope pressed firmly against the chest wall (Figure 224).**

    This technique is similar to that used in the detection of a faint murmur due to aortic regurgitation. Before ruling out the presence of a pericardial friction rub, remember to listen with the patient prone and propped up on his or her elbows. Occasionally this is the only position in which the findings of a friction rub might be heard (Figure 225).

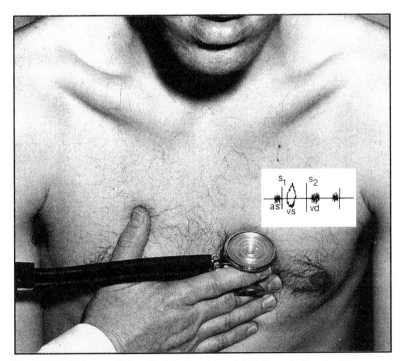

Figure 224: To Hear a Rub — To detect a pericardial friction rub: Use the flat diaphragm of the stethoscope. Listen along the third and fourth left sternal border. Exert firm pressure with the patient sitting upright, breath held in deep expiration. Note three component friction rub:
as = Atrial systolic component.
vs = Ventricular systolic component.
vd = Ventricular diastolic component.
The ventricular systolic component (vs) in the drawing of this patient was loud with a musical quality.

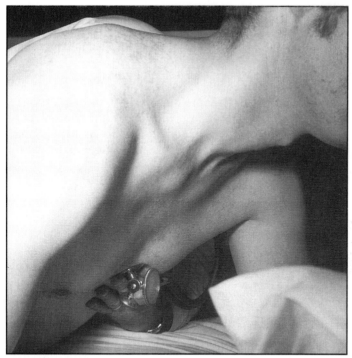

Figure 225: Listening for a Friction Rub — Patient lying on his stomach propped up on his elbows is sometimes the best way to hear a pericardial friction rub. Listen with the diaphragm of the stethoscope pressed firmly at the mid-left sternal border.

- **Another use of this position: Occasionally, a faint aortic diastolic murmur might best or only be heard if the diaphragm of the stethoscope is pressed quite firmly along the third left sternal border — with the patient prone and propped on his or her elbows.**

- **This position is also useful in detecting pericardial effusion (Figure 226).**

Usually when a patient is examined in the supine position and then turns over on his stomach, propped up on his elbows, the heart sounds and murmurs may become louder. (The stethoscope is closer to the heart sounds and murmurs in this position). However, in the case of pericardial effusion of moderate degree, the heart sound may *decrease* in intensity when the patient turns on his stomach (Figures 227, 228 and 229). Presumably this is due to the fact that gravity causes a layer of pericardial fluid to gather between the stethoscope and the heart when the patient is in this position.

This procedure can be particularly helpful in diagnosing moderate to severe effusion. Milder degrees of effusion may not muffle the heart sounds and murmurs. Very severe degrees of pericardial effusion can be clinically suspected without having to turn the patient in this position. Therefore it is in the presence of more moderate degrees of pericardial effusion where this bedside maneuver should be used more frequently as an aid in the clinical diagnosis, which, of course, can be confirmed by echocardiography.

- **Suspect acute pericarditis when a patient says, "I have pain in my chest when I am lying down, but I can get relief if I sit up and get in a certain position."**

It is interesting to observe such a patient who will, on sitting, repeatedly get in the same position, perhaps leaning on a pillow, or on the type of bedside table that extends over the bed. Pain may resume, unfortunately, with only slight changes of position.

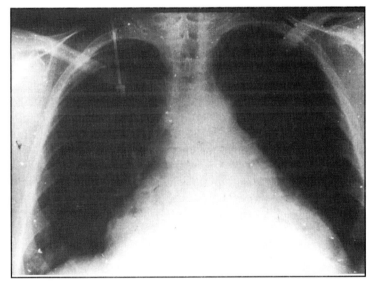

Figure 226: Pericardial Effusion.

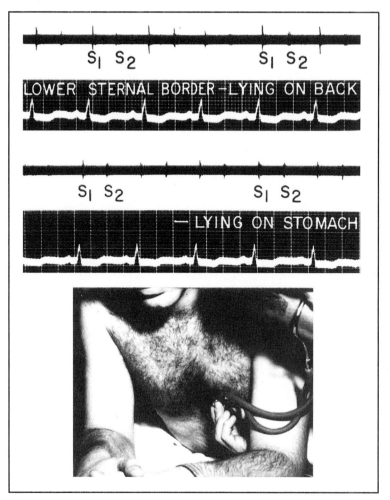

Figure 227: Patient with Pericardial Effusion — Heart sounds (S₁, S₂) become much fainter when he turns from lying flat on his back to his stomach, propped up on his elbows.

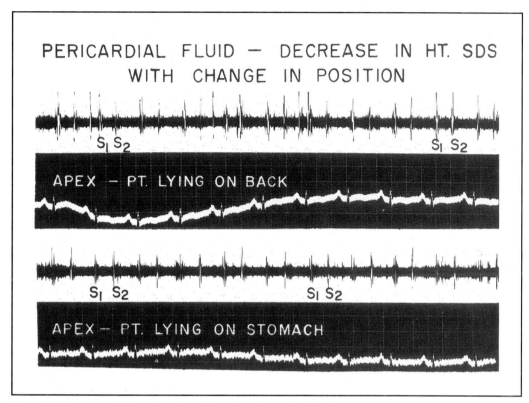

Figure 228: Decrease in Heart Sounds — The patient has pericardial effusion.

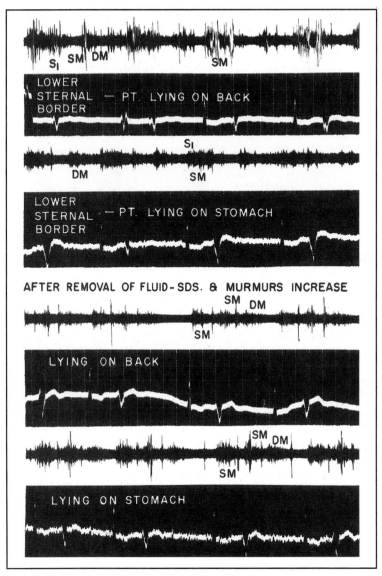

Figure 229: Back to Stomach — Another patient with pericardial effusion. In the top two tracings we see that the heart sounds become fainter when the patient turns from his back to his stomach due to the insulation of the pericardial fluid. After removal of the fluid, the sounds are louder when he is on his stomach (bottom).

Constrictive Pericarditis

- **Pericardial Knock Sound** — The pericardial knock sound of constrictive pericarditis is present in the great majority of patients who have this condition, if one carefully searches for it.

This is a solid cardiac pearl aiding in the diagnosis. The knock sound is present in 90% or more of patients with constrictive pericarditis. The sound occurs in the ventricle during the rapid filling phase of early diastole and is probably produced by blood striking the ventricular walls. It may be misinterpreted as the opening snap of mitral stenosis. However, in timing it occurs later after the second sound than does the opening snap of a tight mitral stenosis, but earlier than the normal physiological third heart sound or ventricular (S_3) gallop.

If one hears a sound thought to be the opening snap of mitral stenosis, listen over the point of maximum impulse of the left ventricle with the patient turned to the left lateral position. If you don't hear a diastolic rumble, you might at first assume that perhaps the bell of the stethoscope is not over the localized spot where a rumble of mitral stenosis would be heard. However, if, on listening over various localized spots and double checking that the bell of the stethoscope is indeed over the point of maximum impulse, you still do not hear a rumble but only the extra sound that could be an opening snap of mitral stenosis, do a "double take." Check the neck veins and if there is definite distention, constrictive pericarditis is the diagnosis. This cardiac pearl has stood the test of time and can provide an immediate diagnostic clue to constrictive pericarditis (Figure 230). The correct diagnosis can be suggested even earlier in the physical examination by examining the jugular venous pulse in the neck, as should be done on examination of every patient.

Poorly appreciated is the fact that pericardial knock sounds can be several rather than single (Figures 231 and 232). Also, pericardial knock sounds can occasionally occur in systole as well as in diastole (Figure 234).

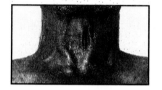 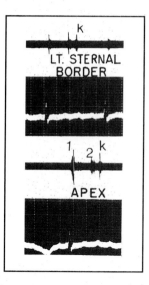 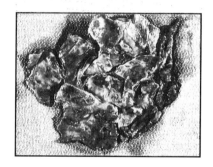

Figure 230: The Clues and the Cause — Distended neck veins (left) plus pericardial knock sound (k) (middle) equals constrictive pericarditis. (Right — pieces of constricting pericardium removed at surgery)

● Rheumatoid arthritis can cause pericardial disease.

Constrictive pericarditis in the United States is usually viral in origin. A number of years ago, tuberculosis was a common cause of constrictive pericarditis, but today this is uncommon, although it does occur. Another, though poorly recognized, cause is rheumatoid arthritis. Pericardial disease due to rheumatoid arthritis can be of varying degrees of severity. Often it is not significant enough to be clinically recognized in life, but is only picked up at autopsy. In other patients, however, it can be severe enough to cause constrictive pericarditis. Recalled is a patient in his 50's who was so cachectic and emaciated that he looked like a patient in the last stages of cancer. He had gained about 70 pounds of weight due to accumulation of edema fluid. Advanced cardiac decompensation was present and none of the medications given were effective in alleviating his symptoms.

His hands showed advanced rheumatoid arthritis, which was the first clue to pay strict attention to the cardiac findings. His neck veins were constantly distended, standing out like fingers over the supraclavicular areas and neck. On auscultation, he had a sound consistent with that of a pericardial knock (Figure 234), which sounds very similar to the opening snap of mitral stenosis, except that it usually occurs a bit later in diastole. He also had bilateral enlargement and tenderness of his breasts, which was presumably due to the digoxin that he was taking.

Surgery to correct his constrictive pericarditis was successful. By one year later he had lost 70 pounds of edema fluid, gained good flesh weight, and was hardly recognizable as the same person that had been evaluated a year before.

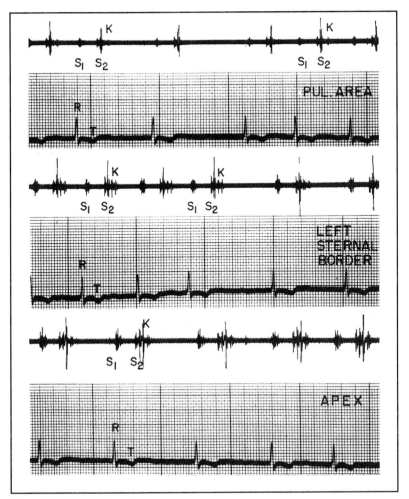

Figure 231: Multiple Knocks.

- **Another pearl:** Pulsus paradoxus can be present with constrictive pericarditis, but it is more likely to occur with cardiac tamponade.

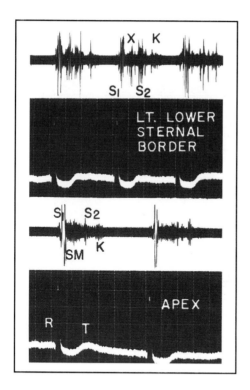

Figure 232: Unusual — Note several knock sounds (K) in diastole and also in systole (X), which is unusual. A systolic murmur (SM) was also present.

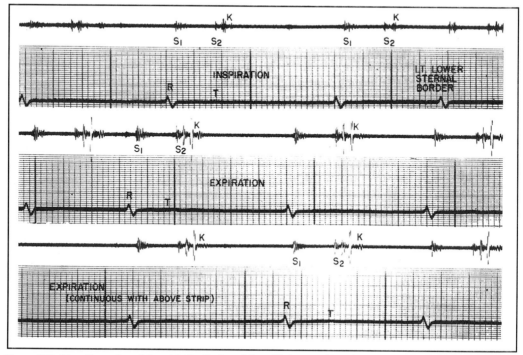

Figure 233: More Examples of Constrictive Pericarditis — Note several knock sounds (k) rather than a single sound. Also this patient's knock sounds are louder in expiration.

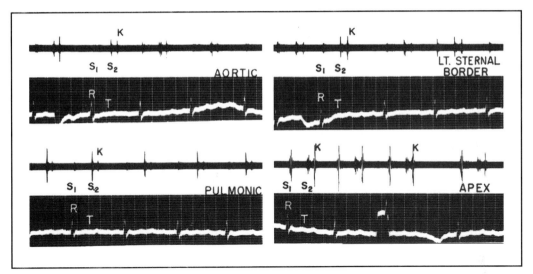

Figure 234: Rheumatoid Arthritis Plus Pericarditis — Note pericardial knock sound (k) heard over the precordium, but best heard over the apex and left sternal border.

- **A patient with early or mild constrictive pericarditis may have a pericardial knock heard *only* on inspiration (Figure 235).**

- **How to differentiate the opening snap of mitral stenosis from the pericardial knock sound of constrictive pericarditis.**

These two sounds can be similar and cause confusion. Here are clues to differentiate them.
1. The first sound in mitral stenosis is usually loud when the opening snap is heard. The first sound associated with the pericardial knock is often not accentuated, although it can be.
2. P_2 is accentuated with mitral stenosis, but not with constrictive pericarditis.
3. The diastolic murmur of mitral stenosis is usually heard over the point of maximum impulse of the left ventricle. A diastolic murmur is hardly ever present with constrictive pericarditis. An exception: Very very rarely, constriction between the left atrium and left ventricle has occurred, resulting in a diastolic murmur.
4. Neck vein distention is characteristic of constrictive pericarditis, but does not usually occur with mitral stenosis.
5. Rheumatic heart disease usually has two valves involved, the aortic and the mitral. This is not so with constrictive pericarditis.

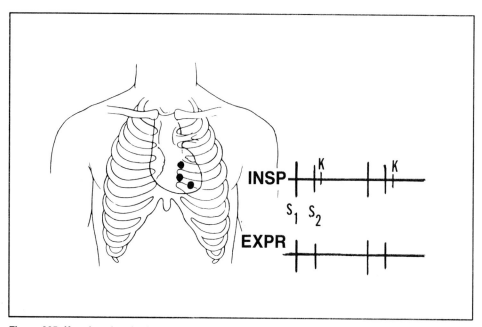

Figure 235: Knock on Inspiration — Early, or mild, constrictive pericarditis. Note pericardial knock sound (k) heard only on inspiration. S_1 = First sound; S_2 = second sound.

Ejection Sounds

In some patients having congenital heart disease, the first heart sound over the pulmonic area and third left sternal border may at first seem to be split. Often, however, this is not splitting, but rather a pulmonary ejection sound occurring in early systole and related to: Congenital valvular pulmonic stenosis, idiopathic dilation of the pulmonary artery or pulmonary hypertension due to ventricular defect, atrial defect, patent ductus, and primary pulmonary hypertension. The pulmonary ejection sound may be well heard in expiration and decrease in intensity with inspiration.

The aortic ejection sound, however, is usually well heard at the apex and also at the aortic area. It does not diminish in intensity with inspiration.

The aortic ejection sound occurs when there is "doming" of the bicuspid valve in early systole. The same holds true for congenital stenosis of the pulmonary valve — the ejection sound occurs with it "doming" in early systole.

- **Rule out a systolic ejection sound when the "first sound" over the pulmonic area seems louder than usual. This may be a pulmonary ejection sound masquerading (or being misinterpreted) as the first sound.**

It is suggested that the term "click" be reserved for the click sounds that occur with mitral valve prolapse, and not used to describe ejection sounds, which are commonly referred to as "aortic ejection click" or "pulmonic ejection click". Rather, use ejection *sound*. This will result in a more orderly, clearer terminology.

- **Differentiating Between Aortic Stenosis and Pulmonic Stenosis — The ejection sound of a bicuspid aortic valve is generally well heard at the apex as well as over the aortic area. It does not alter with respiration. On the other hand, a pulmonic ejection sound from a congenital pulmonic valve stenosis usually localized over the second or third left sternal border, characteristically has an ejection sound that may decrease or even disappear coincident with inspiration. It is generally not heard at the apex as is the rule with a bicuspid aortic stenosis.**

Ejection sounds also can occur in the absence of aortic or pulmonary valve stenosis. A pulmonic ejection sound can occur with a patient having pulmonary hypertension, idiopathic dilatation or aneurysm of the pulmonary artery which in some, and similar to pulmonary valve stenosis, may also increase in intensity coincident with inspiration. An aortic ejection sound may be present with aneurysm of the ascending aorta, and in more advanced degrees of aortic regurgitation.

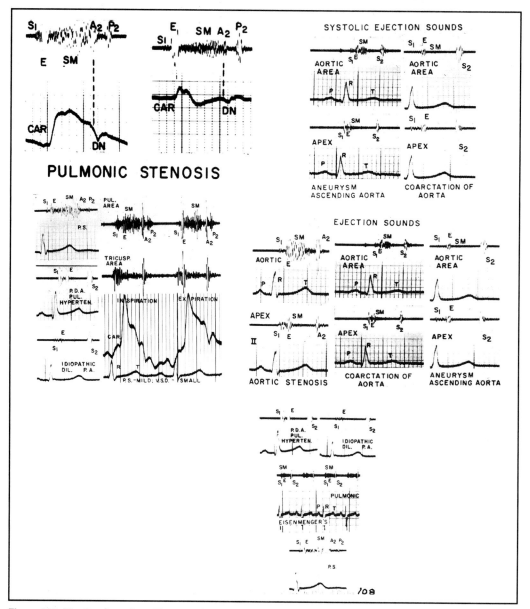

Figure 236: Ejection Sounds — These tracings show a composite of various ejection sounds, both valvular and non-valvular.

266

An aortic ejection sound is a "hallmark" of a congenital bicuspid aortic valve. An early to midsystolic murmur is also usually present, and both the murmur and the ejection sound are heard at the apex as well as over the aortic area. Remember the cardiac pearl — Aortic events are also well heard at the apex.

An ejection sound may be heard with coarctation of the aorta. I had the opportunity to evaluate a number of patients with coarctation referred to the pioneer cardiovascular surgeon, Dr. Robert Gross of Children's Hospital, Boston. His adult patients were worked up at the Peter Bent Brigham Hospital (across the street). I found that a number of these patients had an aortic ejection sound, the etiology of which was at first unclear. Subsequently, it became clear: A congenital bicuspid aortic valve is the most commonly associated congenital defect in patients with coarctation. The aortic ejection sound of the bicuspid valve is the reason for it. Therefore, when we hear an aortic ejection sound in a patient with coarctation of the aorta, the diagnosis of a bicuspid valve is also likely (Figure 237).

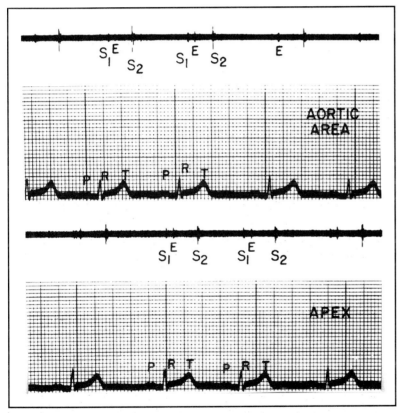

Figure 237: Patient with Coarctation — The ejection sound (E) heard at the apex and aortic area immediately suggests another congenital lesion — a bicuspid aortic valve.

Coarctation of the Aorta

- **The diagnosis of coarctation of the aorta can generally be made by several simple findings: Hypertension in the upper arms, a basal systolic murmur, and decreased or absent femoral arterial pulsations.**

   The basal systolic murmur is usually heard best over the aortic and/or pulmonic areas; since innocent systolic murmurs are frequently present over these areas, the cardiac pearl is that a similar systolic murmur is detected in the supraclavicular areas and in the interscapular region. It is well known that very loud murmurs heard over the front of the chest can be transmitted to the back.

- **What is very helpful with coarctation is that the systolic murmur can be clearly heard over the back even though over the anterior chest it is only of grade 2 or 3 intensity.**

   It is usually a bit fainter over the back, but it can be as loud. The reason for this is that the site of the coarctation, as a rule, is about midway between the front and back of the chest.

   Another etiology of the murmur in the back is the enlarged collateral arteries that are often present with coarctation and some murmurs are actually produced over these vessels.

- **Palpation of the femoral arteries should be a routine part of the physical examination of every patient (Figure 238).**

   An exception to the femoral artery pulsations being weak or absent with coarctation is if the coarctation is associated with severe advanced aortic regurgitation; if so, the femoral pulsations may be normal or even accentuated.

- **How to suspect this: Palpate the femoral pulsation simultaneously with an artery above the coarcted site (radial, brachial, or carotid). The femoral pulsation is weaker. As** a rule, with severe aortic regurgitation alone, the femoral pulsation is better felt than the radial, brachial, or carotid pulsations (Figures 239 and 240).

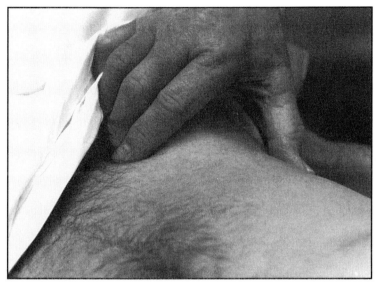

Figure 238: Palpation of the Right Femoral Artery — Palpation of both femoral arteries should be routine in examination of every patient. Some physicians prefer to palpate with the thumb.

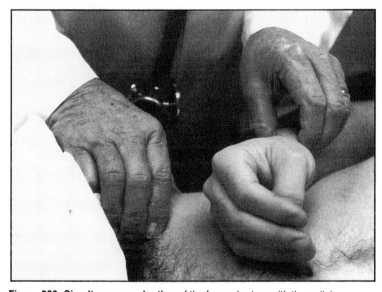

Figure 239: Simultaneous palpation of the femoral artery with the radial.

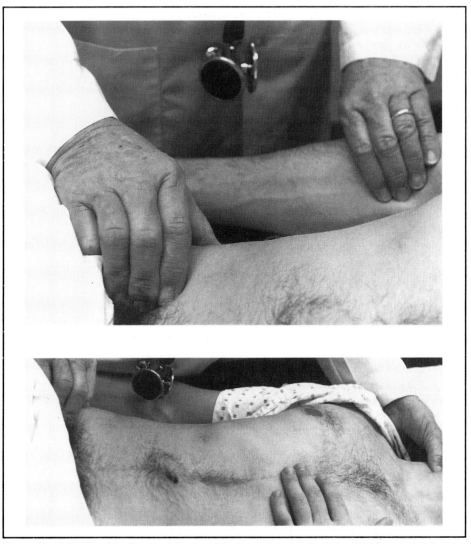

Figure 240: Other Combinations — Palpation of the femoral artery with the brachial (upper photo) and the carotid (lower photo).

Surgical correction is preferably performed in youth and not in middle or older ages. It is of interest that bicuspid congenital aortic valves and congenital cerebral aneurysms may be associated lesions.

Remember, if a patient with coarctation of the aorta has aortic regurgitation with a systolic ejection sound, always suspect an associated congenital bicuspid aortic valve rather than rheumatic etiology of aortic regurgitation (Figure 241).

Palpation of the pulsations of intercostal arteries may be a clue to the diagnosis of coarctation, as exemplified by a nurse in a well known university hospital; she made the initial diagnosis by detecting these pulsations when washing the patient's back.

Rib notching, as noted on x-ray of the chest, occurs as a result of these pulsating intercostal arteries. They are usually felt over the mid and upper back bilaterally.

- **Cardiac pearl: Abdominal aortic coarctation can occur, but is uncommon. Notching of the lower ribs (absent in the upper) may afford a clue.**

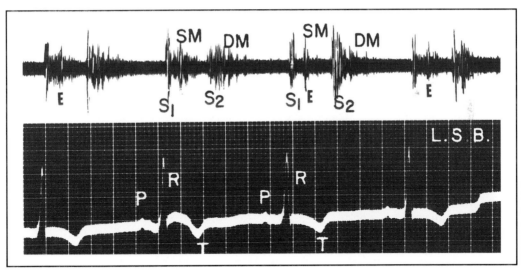

Figure 241: Coarctation of the Aorta Plus Aortic Regurgitation — Note ejection sound (E) in addition to the systolic (SM) and diastolic (DM) murmurs.

Continuous Murmurs

- **All that is continuous is not patent ductus.**

    Dr. William Nelson of the University of South Carolina, Columbia, has had a special interest in continuous murmurs. His list of the possible causes of continuous murmurs is as follows:

    Patent ductus arteriosus
    Aortic pulmonic window
    Truncus I-II-III
    Anomalous origin of left coronary artery from the pulmonary artery
    Accessory coronary artery
    Sinus of Valsalva fistula
    Coronary-arterial fistula
    Systemic arteriovenous fistula
    Pulmonary arteriovenous fistula
    Blalock-Taussig operation
    Potts operation
    Waterston operation
    Coarctation of the aorta
    Coarctation of the pulmonary artery
    Pulmonary thromboembolism
    Arteritis
    Arteriosclerosis obliterans
    Coronary "stenosis"
    Venous hum — neck
    Mammary hum — breast (pregnancy)
    Total anomalous pulmonary venous connection
    Coarctation collaterals
    Bronchial collaterals
        — Truncus-IV
        — "Pseudo-truncus"
        — Tricuspid atresia
        — Severe Tetralogy of Fallot
    Cruveiller-Baumgarten Syndrome

    Murmurs of congenital ventricular septal defect with aortic regurgitation have been called "continuous" and misdiagnosed as patent ductus (Figure 242).

In the past patients were operated upon thinking patent ductus was the lesion, only to find that there was no ductus. The systolic and diastolic murmurs of ventricular defect with aortic regurgitation do not envelop the second heart sound as is typical of the ductus murmur. This distinction can be appreciated with one's stethoscope.

• Arteriovenous Fistula — An arteriovenous communication may be large enough to produce congestive heart failure.

A soldier was admitted to Walter Reed Army Hospital with classic signs of advanced cardiac decompensation. However, at first, no specific etiology could be determined. His diagnosis was that of dilated cardiomyopathy. Careful auscultation over the back (Figures 243 and 244) paid off when listening over a scar over the lower spine and detecting a continuous loud murmur. The scar was the result of a previous lumbar disc operation. An arteriovenous fistula had been created at surgery, which resulted in his heart failure. Following surgical correction of this fistula, his heart returned to normal — another example of a curable type of heart disease.

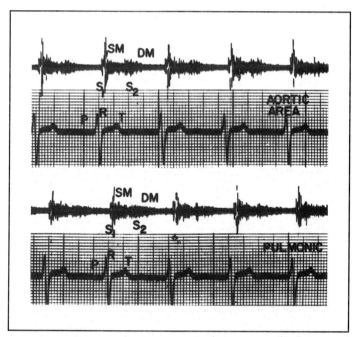

Figure 242: A Patient with Ventricular Septal Defect and Aortic Regurgitation — These murmurs (SM, DM) are often called continuous, and may be misdiagnosed as patent ductus. However, there is the holosystolic (SM) murmur of ventricular defect, plus the aortic diastolic murmur (DM) of aortic regurgitation that tails off immediately after the second sound. The murmurs do not envelop the second sound (S_2), as is characteristic of the ductus murmur.

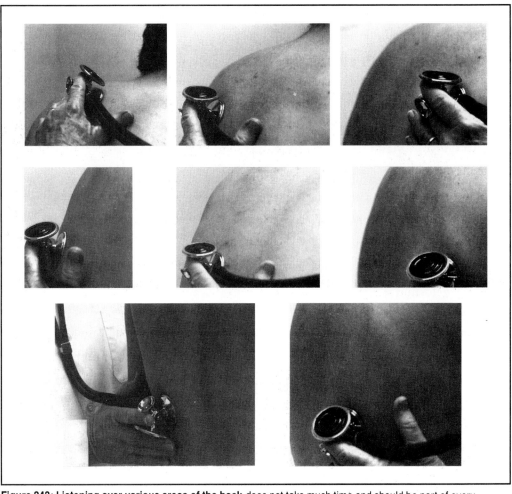

Figure 243: Listening over various areas of the back does not take much time and should be part of every patient's examination. At times it affords a clue to the diagnosis.

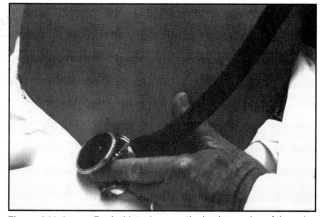

Figure 244: Lower Back: Listening over the lumbar region of the spine.

- **Cardiac Pearl:** Be sure to listen with your stethoscope over every *scar*. The findings may be rewarding (Figure 245).

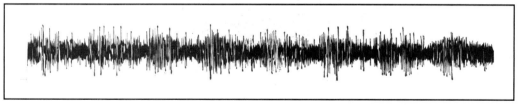

Figure 245: **A-V Fistula** — A continuous murmur of an A-V fistula due to trauma.

- **Cardiac Pearl:** Listen with the stethoscope over areas other than the precordial heart areas.

- **The Osler-Weber-Rendu Syndrome (a pulmonary arteriovenous fistula)** — Careful examination of the lips and buccal membranes may reveal small, reddish-purple telangiectasia which provide an immediate clue to the possible presence of this syndrome. If searched for carefully, a continuous murmur might be detected over an arteriovenous shunt in the lung (Figure 245A).

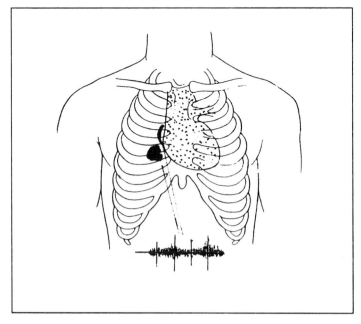

Figure 245A: A patient with Osler-Weber-Rendu syndrome. Note continuous murmur heard along lower right sternal border as shown by area indicated.

Such a lesion can produce clubbing of the fingers and toes and cyanosis. The x-ray and angiography may document one or more lesions that might be amenable to surgical correction. This is another example of a curable type of heart disease.

- **Mammary Hum — A continuous murmur termed mammary hum (bruit) may be heard over the breasts of a new mother, particularly one who is nursing her infant (Figure 246). It can occur over either breast, but if it is heard over the left breast it can be mistaken for a patent ductus or coronary arteriovenous fistula. The mammary hum is a perfectly benign finding and the patient can be reassured concerning it. Pressure over the localized spot of this murmur may eliminate it.**

- **Maternal Souffle — While listening to a pregnant woman's abdomen, particularly in the last trimester of pregnancy, a continuous murmur may be heard. This is a normal, benign finding called maternal souffle (Figure 247).**

This murmur frequently has a musical character, sometimes with a high frequency.

- **A continuous innocent venous hum murmur in the neck is a common finding in children.**

Such a murmur was personally observed in every one of approximately 100 school children 10 to 12 years old when it was carefully searched for using the following technique: The patient should be in the sitting position (the hum's origin is venous blood flow in the jugular vein which empties into the right atrium). On auscultation, the right hand places the bell of the stethoscope over the right supraclavicular fossa; the left hand holds the patient's chin from behind and tilts it upward and to the left. When an optimal position of the neck "on a stretch" is reached, the hum, if present, will be heard (Figure 248).

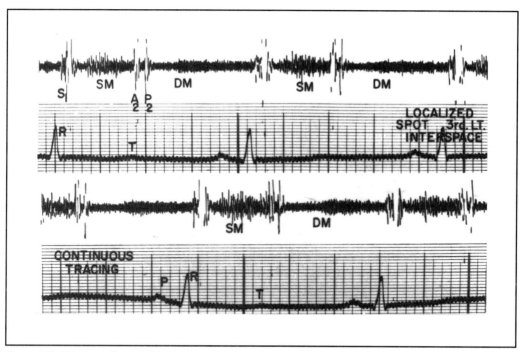

Figure 246: Mammary Hum — This patient was a 24-year-old woman who was breast feeding her baby. Note continuous murmur (SM-DM). The systolic portion of the murmur peaks in midsystole and does not envelop the second sound. The diastolic component is louder in the second half of systole.

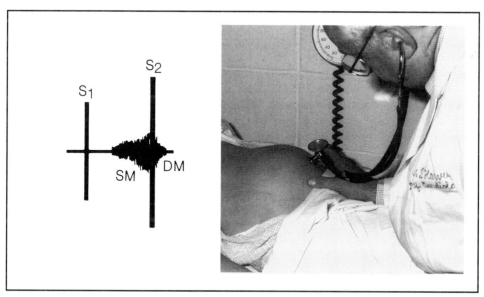

Figure 247: Maternal Souffle — Innocent murmur heard over a mother's abdomen has predominant late systolic component (SM) and faint early diastolic component (DM).

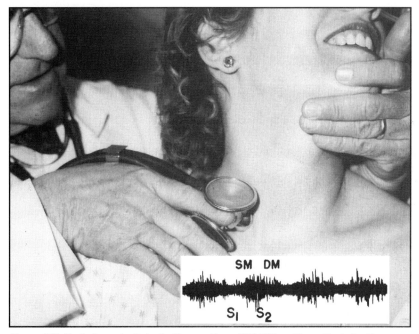

Figure 248: Techniques to Detect a Venous Hum, (SM-DM) — The patient sits. The physician listens with the bell of the stethoscope over the right supraclavicular fossa, while his left hand holds the chin and moves it in the opposite direction and "on a stretch."

It frequently has the character of a continuous loud, low frequency roaring murmur, and it usually can be made to disappear by moving the head to the forward position. Light pressure with the finger over the upper part of the jugular vein will cause the murmur to cease (Figure 249), although uncommonly a high frequency, faint, "whining" continuous murmur remains.

A venous hum is present in conditions associated with a rapid circulation and an increased cardiac output. It is an expected finding in pregnancy, anemia, and hyperthyroidism.

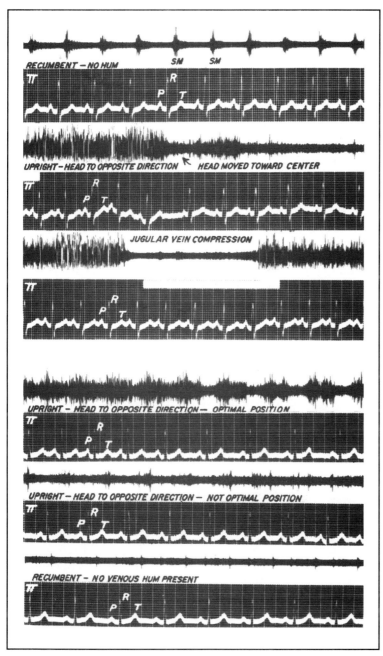

Figure 249: Two Examples of a Venous Hum.

Venous Hum

- **On careful examination of approximately 90 National Football League players, a venous hum was detected in all.**

The frequency of occurrence of a venous hum in these players (ages in their 20's or early 30's) was similar to that of children. Why is this? Remember that the venous hum is probably the result of a degree of normal mild obstruction of venous blood flow in the jugular vein to the right side of the heart, heard with the bell of the stethoscope placed over the supraclavicular fossa, especially when the patient's head is turned to the opposite direction and the neck is on a stretch. Many professional football players are large, muscular men weighing 250 to 300 pounds. They work out with weights and a common result is the development of large neck muscles (Figure 250).

It is interesting to theorize from the armchair that this muscular enlargement produces some degree of pressure on the jugular vein, which in turn results in some insignificant obstruction to blood flow, similar to what occurs when one listens with the bell of the stethoscope over the supraclavicular fossa with the neck "on a stretch" and turned in the opposite direction. The venous hum in the football players, however, could often be heard with the head in the forward position and became much more easily heard and often quite loud when the neck was put on a stretch.

- **A venous hum can be misdiagnosed as patent ductus arteriosus.**

This continuous murmur may be so prominent that it is heard transmitted over the pulmonic area, thereby being mistaken for patent ductus. This is uncommon, but does occur. In fact, in the past, once or twice a year we would have a young patient referred for surgical correction of a ductus. With tongue in cheek we would say these patients could be *medically cured* of a patent ductus by simple pressure with one's index finger or thumb over the jugular vein, thereby eliminating the murmur (Figures 251 and 252).

If routine auscultation in every patient examined includes the neck regions, a venous hum is often readily identified.

- **Hyperthyroidism — The *absence* of a venous hum practically rules out hyperthyroidism.**

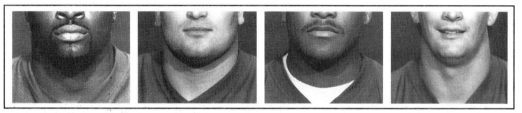

Figure 250: Football Players — Their large muscular necks may make a venous hum more easily heard.

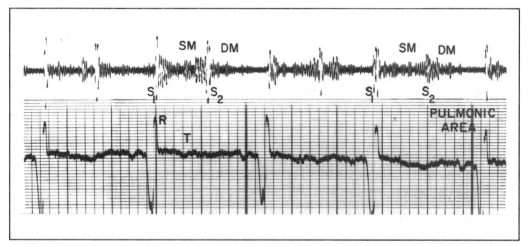

Figure 251: Venous Hum — This venous hum heard over the pulmonic area was misinterpreted as a patent ductus.

Recently, as a coincidence, two patients, each nervous and very hyperactive types, were evaluated within a period of ten days. Each brought up the possibility of hyperthyroidism, but no venous hum was heard. Thyroid studies were normal in both.

● The so-called "thyroid bruit" of hyperthyroidism is usually a venous hum.

Some patients with hyperthyroidism do have a "thyroid bruit" in addition to the venous hum. It is apparently due to the increased blood flow through the vascular thyroid gland. A few patients with hyperthyroids may have a true faint, high frequency, continuous murmur that can be clearly heard after the venous hum is temporarily eliminated by pressure over the jugular vein.

Furthermore, some venous hums not related to thyrotoxicosis can also have a residual high frequency continuous hum when pressure on the jugular vein has eliminated the louder low frequency components.

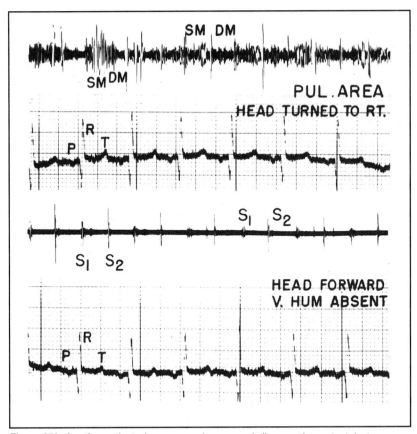

Figure 252: Another patient whose venous hum was misdiagnosed as patent ductus arteriosus. Note that the continuous murmur disappeared when the patient's head was moved to the forward position.

- **In the great majority of patients, the venous hum is best heard over the jugular vein in the *right* supraclavicular fossa. Remember, the head should be turned to the left on a stretch.**

  Occasionally it is better heard over the left supraclavicular fossa with the head turned to the right and on a stretch (Figure 252). As a rule, the patient should be in the sitting position, but occasionally, especially in children, the hum is even heard when they are supine.

- **Even though a venous hum can be loud, the patient usually does not hear it, although one might expect them to.**

  "Never say never." Personally observed was a woman who heard and was bothered by the noise of her loud venous hum. It was definitely proven that she could hear it. She represents the rare example "against the rule."

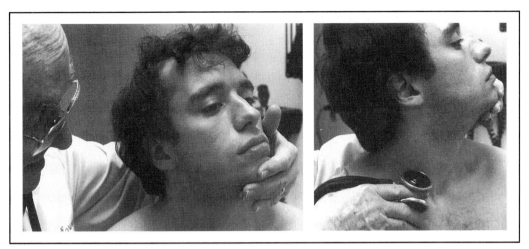

Figure 253: Best Position — The venous hum is usually best heard with the bell of the stethoscope over the *right* supraclavicular fossa, head turned to the left on a stretch.

Dr. Antonio deLeon, Director of Medical Education, St. John Hospital and the University of Tulsa, Oklahoma, tells of a lady who heard a roaring sound when she turned her head to back her car out of the driveway. This apparently was related to her loud venous hum that she heard when she turned her head, putting her neck on a stretch, which accentuated her venous hum (Figure 254).

Recently I was made aware of another patient who had this annoyance. However, despite these exceptions, it is very rare for the patient to hear his or her own venous hum.

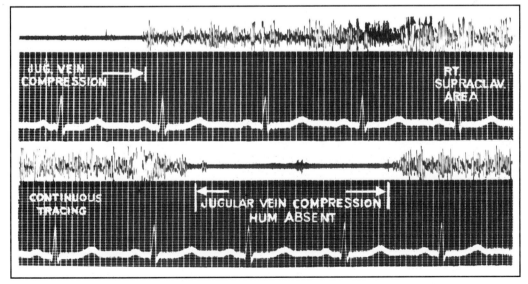

Figure 254: Audible Hum — This middle aged lady could hear her own venous hum. It disappeared with compression on the jugular vein, as shown in the tracing.

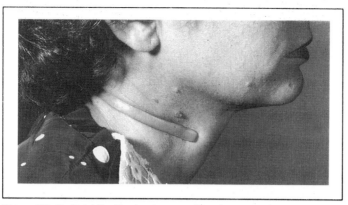

Figure 255: To Quiet the Hum — A rare patient who can actually hear her venous hum. A plastic choker was devised to eliminate the murmur. However, she subsequently decided not to wear it and simply put up with her murmur.

• Bird-like Movements — A clue to the presence of thyrotoxicosis.

A lady of about 70 years of age had no venous hum that could be elicited. She had cervical arthritis to the degree that it was difficult to listen over the right supraclavicular area in the neck with her head turned to the opposite direction, and on a stretch. However, she did have (what my mentor, the late Samuel A. Levine, taught me) quick bird-like movements sometimes apparent with thyrotoxicosis. When asked to sit up from the lying position, she did so very quickly. Most 70-year-old patients would do so slowly and gradually. She also had a quick wit.

• Other subtle "pearls" of thyrotoxicosis: If we ask the patient to sit up and we feel where he or she has been lying it may be warmer than expected, due to the increased metabolism.

Husbands and wives may get into arguments because one wants a lot of bed covers and the other doesn't want any. Guess which one has the increased metabolism? Menopause, of course, could be a "red herring".

Another interesting patient: A young boy was referred for evaluation because his muscle and bone development was definitely impaired. He had had a congenital patent ductus repaired about a year before. The question was, could his problem be related to his congenital heart disease, now surgically corrected, or did he have some additional congenital problems? Neither of these possibilities proved to be present. He appeared to be about six years of age, but actually was nine years old. It was summer time and his hospital room was comfortable, although there was no air conditioning. It was noticed that he was sleeping with his socks on and under blankets. He stated he always did so. This was now a clue to his problem: He had primary hypothyroidism. With thyroid medication, "he grew like a weed", as was subsequently reported by his physician.

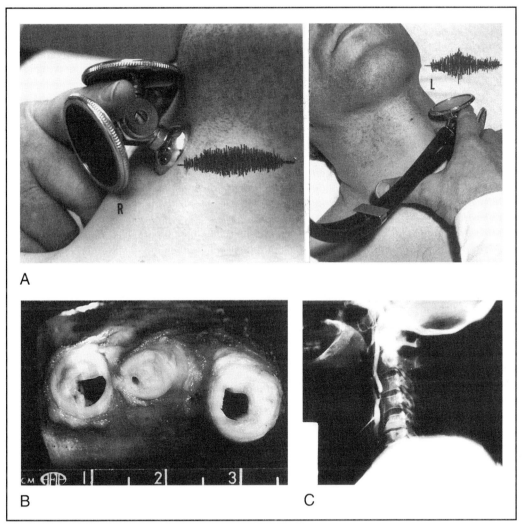

Figure 256 A, B, C: Occlusion — This patient had bilateral carotid artery occlusion producing a continuous murmur on both sides. R = right neck, L = left neck. Note pathology of carotid artery occlusive disease (256B) and carotid arteriogram (256C) demonstrating occlusion.

- **Listen over the neck in every patient (Figure 256).**

     A physician in his sixties had several episodes of syncope. He had a history of a previous myocardial infarction. Our first thought was that a ventricular arrhythmia, transient tachycardia or fibrillation would explain the syncope. Instead, on physical examination a loud continuous murmur was heard over both carotid arteries and each proved to be 90% occluded (Figure 256). Endarterectomy solved this problem. The lesson we learned: Listen over the neck in every patient.

     Figure 257 illustrates how valuable information can be quickly obtained by listening over the neck. The bell chest piece should be used in order to make an air seal; this particularly applies to listening over the suprasternal notch (Figures 258 and 259). Figure 260 illustrates the use of the bell over the left and right supraclavicular areas where both "innocent" and "guilty" (significant) murmurs can be heard.

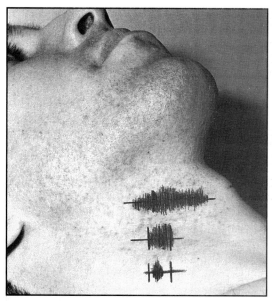

Figure 257: Type of murmurs (bruits) heard in the neck, not including innocent venous hum: Top: Continuous murmur of obstruction. Middle: Carotid artery occlusion of mild to moderate degree. Lower: Short early to mid (innocent) systolic murmur heard in supraclavicular fossa bilaterally.

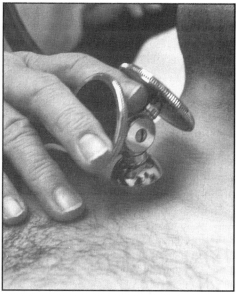

Figure 258: Use the bell of the stethoscope to listen over the suprasternal notch.

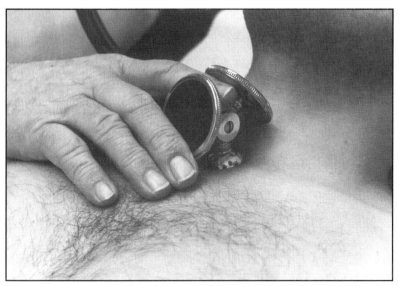

Figure 259: Listening Over the Suprasternal Notch — Note the bell chest piece snugly fits in this area, making the necessary air seal. Large bell or diaphragm chest pieces do not accomplish this.

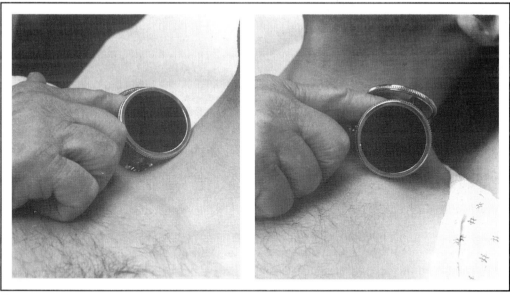

Figure 260: Listening with the Bell of the Stethoscope Over the Right and Left Supraclavicular Areas — Murmurs of aortic stenosis are transmitted to these areas and are heard equally well on the left and right sides. Innocent venous hums are found here. Have the patient sit, listen in the supraclavicular area with head on a stretch. Short early to mid systolic murmurs are heard over these areas in approximately 25% of young children and teenagers. These short murmurs (bruits) can also be heard in adults. We have also found these innocent findings in athletes such as professional football players.

Patent Ductus Arteriosus

- **Typical Murmur** — The typical continuous murmur of patent ductus arteriosus *envelops* the second heart sound (Figure 261). If the murmur does *not* envelop the second sound, although sounding continuous, this may be a clue that it is due to a cause other than patent ductus.

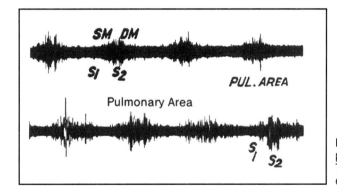

Figure 261: Patent Ductus — Two patients with patent ductus arteriosus. The typical machinery murmur (SM-DM) envelops the second sound (S$_2$).

    An example of this diagnostic trap was a teenage girl referred to our hospital by a well known cardiologist for surgical correction of her ductus. This was at a time when cardiac catheterization was a new procedure and the present day highly technical diagnostic procedures had not been developed. Cardiac catheterization had reportedly been diagnostic of patent ductus. A continuous murmur was heard over the pulmonic area and third left sternal border, which appeared to confirm this diagnosis. To everyone's surprise, at surgery no ductus was present. Instead, the patient had a ventricular septal defect with aortic regurgitation. Her murmur was holosystolic (pansystolic), but peaked in mid-systole rather than enveloping the second sound. The diastolic component was decrescendo after the second sound.

    On review of the literature, we found a case report of a ventricular septal defect associated with aortic regurgitation. The author stated that, clinically, one could not tell the difference between a murmur due to this congenital lesion and one due to patent ductus. The case report contained a figure depicting that patient's murmur. The configuration of the murmur was practically identical to our patient's and did *not* envelop the second sound. Although the author of the case report concluded that one could not clinically differentiate this lesion from patent ductus, we confirmed the important pearl that the typical continuous murmur of patent ductus *envelops* the second sound.

- **The continuous murmur of a large patent ductus is generally loud and of low frequencies, with so-called "eddy" sounds. A palpable continuous thrill is generally present (Figure 262).**

    If one listens to the patient or to a high fidelity recording, these eddy sounds at first might be interpreted as extraneous non-cardiac sounds, or artifacts in the recording; they are, however, the real thing.

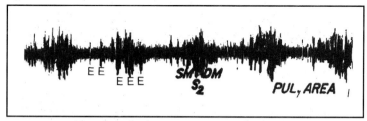

Figure 262: **Another patient** with patent ductus arteriosus. The continuous machinery murmur (SM-DM) envelops the second sound (S$_2$). Eddy sounds (E) are heard with large ducti.

- **Murmurs from small caliber patent ducti are often faint and of higher frequencies. Firm pressure with the diaphragm of one's stethoscope on the chest wall is helpful and often necessary to isolate this murmur.**

- **A very faint continuous murmur from a small patent ductus may become louder and more easily heard by using the isometric handgrip maneuver (Figures 263 and 264).**

    Unless the continuous murmur envelops the second sound, do not call it patent ductus. This difference can easily be detected with the stethoscope.

- **Another cardiac pearl: There are about 30 causes of so-called continuous murmur; thus, "all that is continuous is not patent ductus." (See page 272). Also, "all that rumbles is not mitral stenosis."**

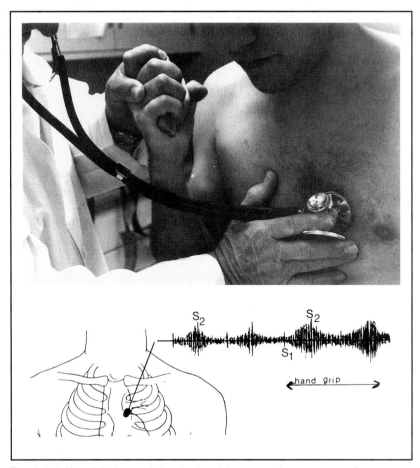

Figure 263: Use of the isometric hand grip to bring out continuous murmur of patent ductus.

Sometimes the continuous murmur of patent ductus is heard louder over the third left sternal border rather than the pulmonic area (Figure 265). However, carefully check out such a patient to make sure there isn't another cause for the continuous murmur, such as coronary arteriovenous fistula, which can produce a murmur over the third or fourth sternal border.

Murmurs from medium sized ducti may have both high and low frequencies, averaging grade 3 or 4, and usually are easily heard on auscultation. These murmurs are loudest over the pulmonic area. We have used the analogy of a pipe organ in the church — the larger pipes have such low frequencies that the room seems to vibrate, while the small pipes produce the melodic high frequency sounds.

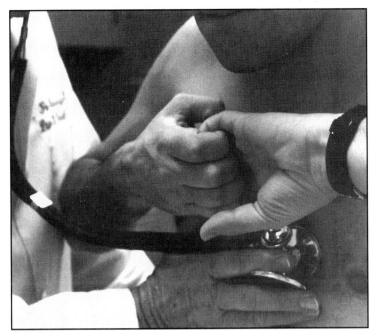

Figure 264: A variant of the hand grip maneuver.

- **Patent Ductus with Pulmonary Hypertension — If pulmonary hypertension develops, this is a serious complication.**

The continuous patent ductus murmur enveloping the second sound may not be present. Instead, the second heart sound becomes accentuated due to the loud pulmonic valve closure, and is closely split. (This may be easily palpated.) An ejection sound may be prominent and only a systolic murmur may be present; or there may be no systolic murmur but a loud diastolic murmur of pulmonary insufficiency may be present. Both the systolic and diastolic murmur, formerly loud, may now be faint (Figures 266 and 267).

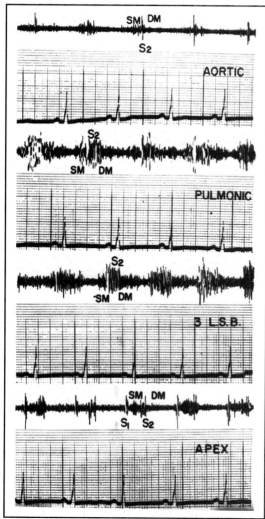

Figure 265: An Exception — Although most continuous murmurs (SM-DM) of patent ductus are best heard over the pulmonic area, occasionally they are louder over the third left sternal border.

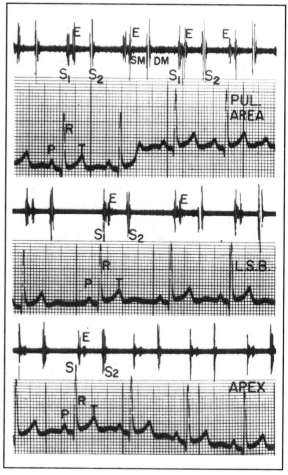

Figure 266: Faint Murmurs in Presence of Patent Ductus and Pulmonary Hypertension — Note absence of continuous murmur enveloping second sound (S_2). A prominent ejection sound (E) and a very loud closely split second sound are present. The systolic (SM) and diastolic (DM) murmurs are faint.

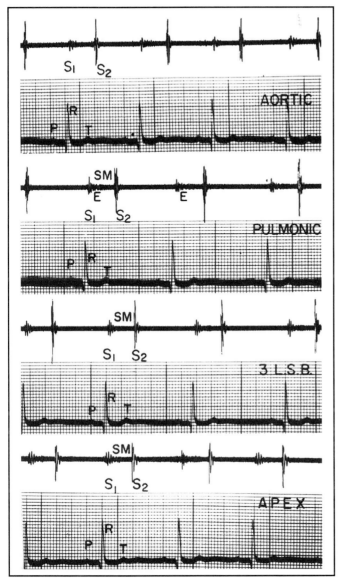

Figure 267: Another example of patent ductus with pulmonary hypertension. No continuous murmur. Note ejection sound (E) and faint systolic murmur (SM).

Electrocardiography

- **Normal Variants:** The absence of an S_4 or S_3 gallop may be helpful in evaluation of a patient who has findings on the ECG suspicious for coronary disease, myocarditis, or cardiomyopathy (dilated or hypertrophic).

I recall a young patient, a talented rookie of one of the major league baseball teams. Because of an electrocardiogram, he had been diagnosed as having either coronary artery disease, myocarditis, or cardiomyopathy. He had some elevation of ST segments and nonspecific ST and T-wave changes, including inversion of the T-waves in the left precordial leads. The patient was referred to me for evaluation.

On questioning this young, healthy-appearing athlete of about 22 years of age, no history could be elicited of any symptoms or signs of heart disease other than the findings on the electrocardiogram, which the patient had with him and presented for review. The physical examination revealed no abnormality whatsoever. It was reasoned that if the patient had either coronary artery disease, myocarditis, or cardiomyopathy producing these findings on electrocardiogram, he should at least have an S_4, and possibly an S_3 gallop, detected on auscultation of the heart (Figures 268 and 269). However, with careful search no extra sound was present. Using this finding of absent gallop, together with a completely negative cardiovascular evaluation, it was suggested to the management of his baseball team that these findings were a variant of normal, particularly since the ST segment elevation and the ST and T-wave changes noted on his ECG are known to occur in healthy people (Figure 270). We recommended that he be allowed to play baseball. The patient did so and I closely followed his performance as reported in the sports pages. He played on his team and had no problem.

About 15 years later, I received a telephone call from him and he asked if I remembered him. I told him that indeed I did. He said that he was in an Emergency Room in a midwestern town and had been diagnosed as having an acute heart attack. His electrocardiogram was described to me via telephone and it was the same as that when I originally saw him. On careful questioning, he had no symptoms consistent with coronary disease. He was therefore sent home.

On another occasion, he telephoned me about an insurance exam he had undergone. The company was reluctant to issue a policy because of the ECG findings. It was related to the officials of the company that these were normal variants and that the patient had no evidence of coronary disease at the time of my evaluation, and showed the same identical electrocardiographic changes.

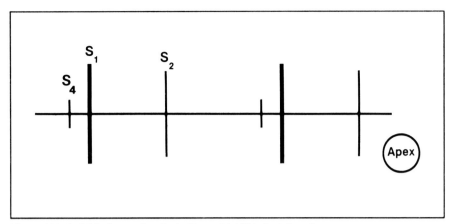

Figure 268: Atrial Gallop — A patient with an atrial (S_4) diastolic gallop.

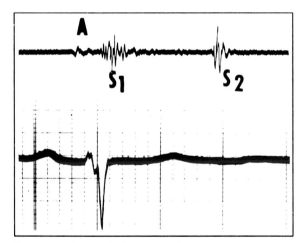

Figure 269: Another Gallop — A patient with coronary artery disease. Note atrial gallop (A) before first sound (S_1).

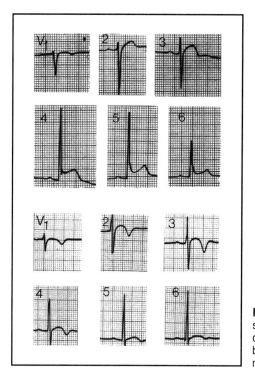

Figure 270: Two Professional Athletes — Note S-T segment elevation and T wave inversions in both. These changes of early repolarization represent a normal variant but can be misdiagnosed as coronary heart disease, myocarditis, or cardiomyopathy.

- **Cardiac Pearl:** In the case of this young baseball player, it was the *absence* of the finding of an atrial (S_4) gallop and/or ventricular (S_3) gallop that supported the clinical impression that his ECG changes were those of early repolarization, a normal variant, and not those of heart disease. Therefore he was able to play and was not deprived of the lucrative salary paid to professional baseball players.

- When one sees straightening of the ST segment producing a right degree angle (as one might see particularly in the left precordial leads and the limb leads), some might refer to this finding as a "nonspecific change". Actually, a common etiology is coronary artery disease (Figure 271).

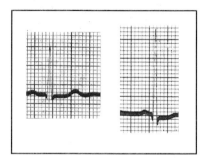

Figure 271: Non-Specific Changes — Two patients having non-specific S-T and T wave change in Lead V₆. Note S-T segment is strengthened coming off the R wave at approximately a 90° angle.

I learned this cardiac pearl from the late George Burch of Tulane.

A misdiagnosis of old anterior myocardial infarction can be made in a patient having a long asthenic chest build and a "tear drop" heart (Figure 272). Electrode placement, even though in the correct interspace, is the culprit. Place the chest electrodes one or one and one half interspaces lower and the normal progression of R wave (rather than slow) may result.

As another case in point, very recently I evaluated a patient who had been previously examined in another medical facility. She had a photocopy of her electrocardiogram (shown in Figure 273), which was normal; however, it is a technically poor tracing as evidenced by the irregular artifact present in each of the 12 leads. This type of tracing can be prevented, or corrected, by paying attention to the following (Figure 274):

a) Make sure there is plenty of electrode paste
b) Check the connections to insure that they are not loose
c) Make sure the electrodes are clean.
d) Is the patient relaxed? If the muscles are tense, artifact can result. The patient can be told how to relax his or her muscles.
e) Are the patient's ankles pressing against the end of the examining table with the feet hanging over? If so, have the patient move upward on the table.
f) Make sure the electrode is positioned over the brachial artery where its pulsation moves the electrode.
g) Repeat the electrocardiogram, if necessary, to get a "good technical tracing."

Practically everyone who has taken a large number of electrocardiograms on patients has inadvertently reversed limb leads in lead 1. Immediate recognition of this mistake can be seen in the tracing, as shown in Figure 275 with inversion of the P-wave and QRS complex — a mirror image of the complex when the electrodes are correctly placed. Always double check for correct attachment of the electrodes when first attaching them and *also when removing them.*

Do you have trouble with chest electrodes falling off? Not uncommonly, precordial electrodes may not stick to the hairy chest of a patient (Figure 276). Often all that is needed to correct this is to put extra paste or gel on the chest and with one's index and/or middle finger, mat down the chest hairs — the electrodes may now hold. Remember to smooth the hairs down on the skin *with the fingers.* Shaving the chest hair, I learned, has been used, at times, but usually is not necessary. Of course, some modern adhesive electrodes stick to the chest skin quite well.

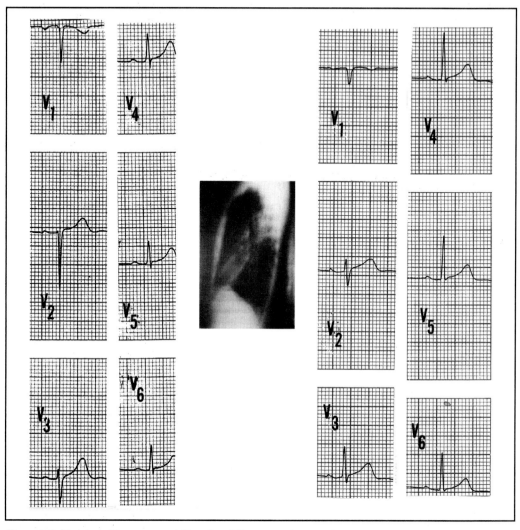

Figure 272: Electrode Placement and "Tear Drop" Heart — Left: Note slow progression of R wave V_1 to V_4, which has been read as consistent with old myocardial infarction. Right: Electrodes placed 1 or 1 ½ interspaces lower show normal progression of R wave. A "tear drop" heart may cause this misdiagnosis. Middle: Note long narrow silhouette of heart on lateral x-ray.

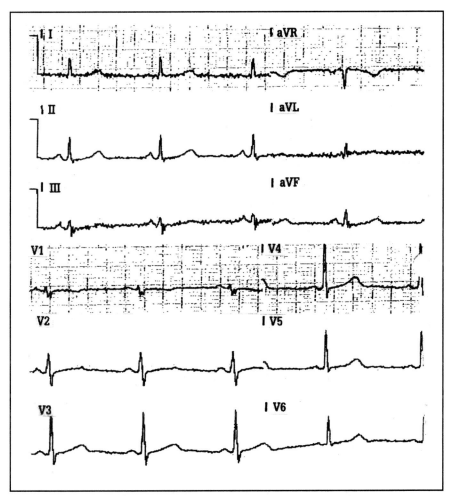

Figure 273: Technically Poor Tracing — This can generally be avoided or eliminated with good simple technique of taking an electrocardiogram.

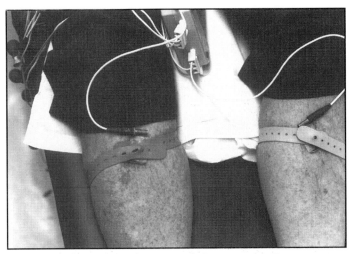

Figure 274: Cause of Artifacts — A technically poor ECG tracing may have artifacts caused by faulty application or preparation of the electrode, or poor relaxation of the patient.

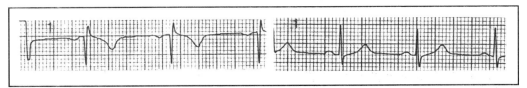

Figure 275: Reversed Leads — Lead 1, right and left arm leads of ECG inadvertently reversed (left tracing). Note negative P wave and mirror image of complex when the limb leads are correct (right tracing). Always double check the lead wires when removing them. In this way the error is promptly detected.

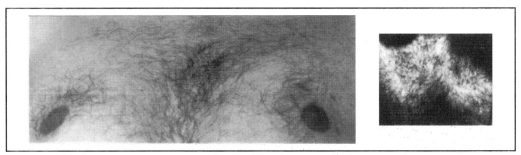

Figure 276: A hairy chest can cause electrodes to fall off, especially a chest such as the one on the right.

Echocardiography

- **Echocardiography is one of the great advances in the diagnosis of cardiovascular disease. However, there is also misuse — Echocardiography is often unnecessary or used for the wrong purpose.**

Personally observed have been requests for a color Doppler echocardiogram and on the request sheet under "Reason for Request" was written "Question murmur." I have been told of similar situations in other echocardiographic laboratories. Sad, but true.

One's stethoscope is the obvious and accurate answer to determining the presence and cause of most murmurs. The aforementioned Reason for Request emphasizes the great need in medicine today to emphasize the *basics* of cardiovascular evaluation, the Five Finger approach, which includes a careful detailed history and physical examination, electrocardiogram, x-ray and simple laboratory tests that can be done in the physician's office or at the bedside. We need to bring the *patient* from the "back burner" up to the front.

- **Overdiagnosis and Underdiagnosis by Echocardiography — Some patients are diagnosed as having mitral valve prolapse because of misinterpretation of the echocardiogram.**

We have personally seen a number of such patients. If a careful clinical search for auscultatory findings of mitral valve prolapse fails to find any evidence of mitral valve prolapse, repeat echocardiogram may also fail to show mitral valve prolapse. A recent example was a 16-year-old high school football player who was evaluated because of a question as to whether he should play. History revealed that the echocardiogram taken by his physician was quoted as "showing mitral valve prolapse."

On physical examination, the patient was entirely asymptomatic and all findings were normal. When listening for auscultatory findings consistent with mitral valve prolapse, none were found. The echocardiogram was repeated at our institution with instructions to take extra time to search for any possibility of prolapse; the echocardiogram was completely normal. This made the decision about playing football quite easy.

- **Overdiagnosis** — At times, too much can be read into an echocardiogram, which can be confusing to the physician. For example, the color Doppler echocardiograph may report the presence of tricuspid regurgitation and/or pulmonary regurgitation when there is no clinical evidence of this, and it does not represent any significance whatsoever as determined from a careful total cardiovascular examination. It should be stated in the report that these findings are frequently present and may be of no importance if the clinical evaluation of the patient reveals no evidence of these conditions.

Too often the report of the presence of these conditions in the absence of any clinical evidence, leads the physician who is not familiar with echocardiography to think that there is significant pathology of the valves; unnecessary anxiety is thereby created for the patient and physician, leading to additional unnecessary and expensive tests.

The same was true of electrocardiography in its earlier days. The late Frank Wilson of the University of Michigan, along with his colleague Franklin Johnston, were instrumental in teaching electrocardiography directly or indirectly to hundreds of thousands of physicians over several decades. Physicians went to the "Mecca" in Ann Arbor, Michigan, to learn electrocardiography from these masters. I was one of them. I heard Dr. Wilson speak on several occasions, and he cautioned us physicians to be careful not to overinterpret the electrocardiogram, since he was aware of the problems that resulted when this was done. He stressed that the electrocardiogram should be part of the total clinical evaluation of a patient. The same problems exist today with the overinterpretation of the echocardiogram.

Ebstein's Anomaly

Ebstein's Anomaly (Figure 277) is a congenital downward displacement of the tricuspid valve into the right ventricle, thereby producing an atrialization of the ventricle. At times, the tricuspid valve is lace-like and portions of it can be matted to the right ventricular wall.

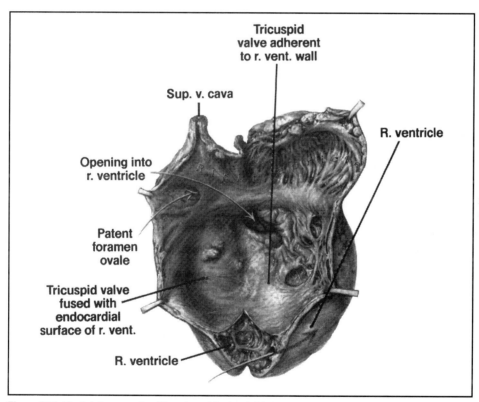

Figure 277: Ebstein's anomaly of the tricuspid valve. With Ebstein's anomaly there is usually a downward displacement of the tricuspid valve which may be adherent to the right ventricular wall. An inefficient right atrium and ventricle results.

- **The second component (tricuspid valve closure) of the first sound may be louder than the first component (mitral valve closure). Normally, the mitral component is the louder (Figures 278 and 279).**

   Atrial septal defect is another congenital anomaly where the tricuspid component may be louder.

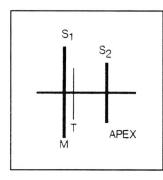

Figure 278: Normal — Mitral valve closure (M) of the first sound (S₁) is louder than tricuspid (T).

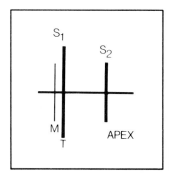

Figure 279: Ebstein's Anomaly — Tricuspid valve closure component of first sound may be louder than the mitral component.

- **Another cardiac pearl about Ebstein's that is very seldom appreciated is that a holosystolic murmur heard over the apex can increase in intensity with inspiration (Figure 280).**

   At first thought, this finding seems to be opposite in that, being over the so-called mitral apical area, the murmur should decrease (Figure 281). However, the clinical pearl of the murmur getting louder holds true because the tricuspid valve in Ebstein's can be at the apex (as well as along the left sternal border) and therefore the murmur characteristically increases with inspiration, indicating tricuspid regurgitation (Figure 282).

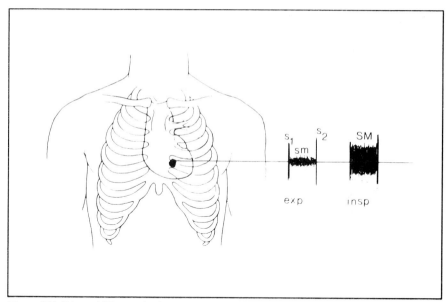

Figure 280: Tricuspid Regurgitation — Ebstein's anomaly. Listening at the lower left sternal border (tricuspid area). Note increase in systolic murmur (SM) with inspiration. In some, this increase is also present at the apex.

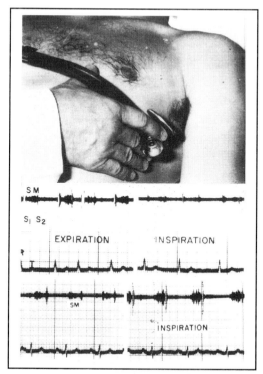

Figure 281: Sign of Ebstein's — The holosystolic murmur of mitral regurgitation should decrease in intensity over the mitral area (top); however, when a holosystolic murmur increases in intensity over this area (bottom), always consider the possibility of Ebstein's anomaly.

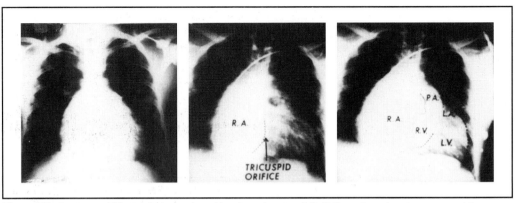

Figure 282: Anatomy of Ebstein's Anomaly — Note large heart on left. At times these hearts can resemble a "water bottle" configuration. The holosystolic murmur of this patient was best heard at the *apex* and it became louder with inspiration, rather than decreasing over the mitral area, as would mitral regurgitation. However, as shown in the middle and right panels above, the location of the tricuspid valve is actually at the location of the usual mitral valve.

Myxoma

- **Most Common Site** — An atrial myxoma is most likely to occur in the left atrium (Figures 283 and 284). Next most common is in the right atrium.

  However, a myxoma can occur in more than one chamber, such as an atrium and a ventricle or in both atria or both ventricles. It is, therefore, important to make a search to rule out the presence of this tumor in more than one place.

- **Surgical Removal** — A myxoma, such as one occurring in the left atrium, can be successfully removed at surgery and without complications such as emboli.

  Some of these tumors are friable and at surgery can break up and embolize to the brain or other areas of the body. In the past this has been a significant problem; however, techniques today accomplish the removal generally without complications. The prognosis following successful removal at surgery is excellent; longer follow ups also show that recurrence of the tumor is not likely.

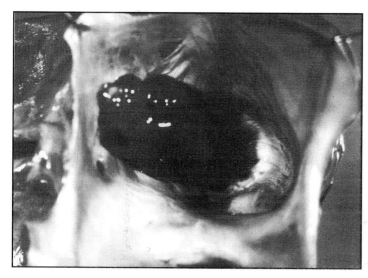

Figure 283: Left atrial myxoma.

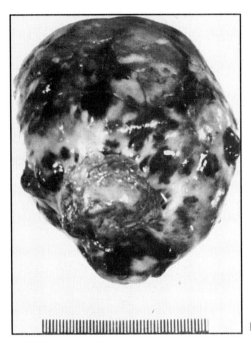

Figure 284: Another left atrial myxoma removed at surgery.

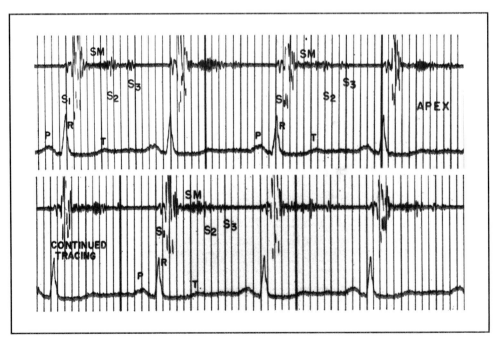

Figure 285: Myxoma of Left Atrium — An Unexpected Finding at Surgery for Supposed Mitral Stenosis — Note similarity to mitral stenosis. The first sound (S1) is loud. The third sound (S_3) is fainter than the usual opening snap of mitral stenosis, and it varies in intensity. The systolic murmur (SM) varies in intensity and position in systole.

- **Atrial Myxoma or Mitral Stenosis? An atrial myxoma can mimic the findings of mitral stenosis (Figure 285). A sound occurring when the tumor moves and strikes the mitral orifice can simulate that of an opening snap.**

However, a change in the timing of this sound after the second sound is consistent with left atrial myxoma, whereas the opening snap of mitral stenosis remains constant. Also, there may be an intermittent change in the intensity of a systolic murmur and/or a diastolic rumble of atrial myxoma, which would not be the case with rheumatic mitral stenosis.

- **Murmur of Atrial Myxoma — Sometimes the diastolic rumble of atrial myxoma can have transient presystolic accentuation.**

A presystolic murmur may occur when the patient's body is in one position and not in another position. The same may hold for the earlier diastolic murmur occurring after the tumor sound, which occurs in early to mid-systole. Atrial myxoma usually represents a curable form of heart disease.

- **Subtle Clues to Atrial Myxoma**

A recent evaluation of a man in his early forties is worthy of description. He was relatively asymptomatic, although on occasion when he changed position, such as getting out of bed, he might feel a bit dizzy. The first clue to his diagnosis came from the electrocardiogram, which was shown in the conference room before we went to see the patient. It showed definite left atrial enlargement by the configuration of the P-wave in lead V_1 (Figure 286). His x-ray, also seen before examining the patient, showed some straightening of the left cardiac silhouette and a density along the right border, which would be consistent with an enlarged left atrium.

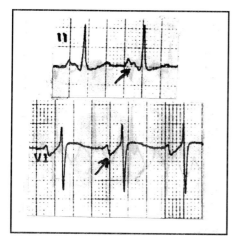

Figure 286: Left atrial enlargement — Note P waves (arrow) on ECG, Leads 2 and V_1.

In this patient, who was essentially asymptomatic, these were enough clues to search with utmost care for some lesion causing left atrial enlargement. He had a detailed cardiac auscultation and at first there were no clues pointing to mitral valve involvement. However, on turning the patient to the left lateral position and listening over the point of maximal impulse, what had first appeared to be a somewhat prolonged first sound proved to be consistent with an extremely short presystolic murmur; then, in another localized spot in this same position, an extra sound was heard in diastole. The sound occurred a bit later than the usual opening snap of mitral stenosis and earlier than a normal third heart sound or S_3 gallop. It had the timing of a pericardial knock of constrictive pericarditis. However, there was no evidence of constrictive pericarditis.

Putting the several simple features together: a short presystolic murmur, a sound occurring in early diastole with the timing of a myxoma (the same timing as a constrictive pericarditis knock), a history of mild dizziness on occasion, left atrial enlargement by electrocardiogram and x-ray, the diagnosis of a left atrial myxoma was suspected and confirmed on echocardiography.

At surgery, a very large left atrial myxoma was successfully removed; the surgeon stated that it was so large that one might wonder how the blood was able to get around such a large obstructing lesion.

- **Syncope from Right Atrial Myxoma — Although syncope can occur in a patient who has rheumatic tricuspid stenosis, this symptom is much more common in patients who have a right atrial myxoma, which can be misdiagnosed as rheumatic tricuspid stenosis.**

The myxoma can temporarily occlude the tricuspid valve orifice and result in dizziness and/or syncope.

- **Dizziness — In a patient having dizziness or syncope, always consider the possibility of a myxoma of either the left or right atrium.**

- **Dizziness or Syncope with Valvular Stenosis — Stenosis of any of the four heart valves can produce these sympoms. However, the closer a diseased valve is to the brain, the more likely it is to cause dizziness or syncope; therefore suspect first the aortic valve.**

Prosthetic Valves

- **Multiple Systolic Sounds** — **Following a valve replacement utilizing the Starr-Edwards ball valve, numerous systolic sounds can be heard which may simulate the rolling of dice on a hard surface or the flipping of a stick on a picket fence (Figure 287).**

These extra sounds can occur in systole as with an aortic valve replacement; the ball "jiggles" at the top of the cage during systole and this produces these multiple sounds. This can be observed on angiography. These same sounds can also be heard in diastole when the artificial valve is in the mitral position; they occur when the ball strikes the end of the cage at the approximate time of the rapid filling phase of the left ventricle in diastole. These sounds are the result of the ball rolling in the cage; there are fewer and fainter rolling sounds in the mitral position than when the valve is in the aortic position. These extra sounds are usually a normal finding and should not cause concern.

- **Porcine Valve** — **An early to midsystolic murmur, usually Grade 2 or 3, is a normal finding following successful valve replacement with a porcine valve. (Figure 288).**

- **Prosthetic valve sounds are sometimes loud enough that the patient can hear them, especially at night or other times when everything is quiet. Sometimes other members of the family also can hear the sounds.**

The first prosthetic valve was implanted by Dr. Charles Hufnagle of Georgetown University Medical Center. He placed this valve in the first portion of the descending aorta (there was no heart-lung pump available at that time). The sounds of this valve, which was made of the same plastic material as one's toothbrush handle, produced loud clicking sounds, and the physicians and surgeons were concerned that these sounds might be a serious annoyance to the patient. The patients were aware of the sounds, but became quite used to them, similar to adapting to a clock ticking.

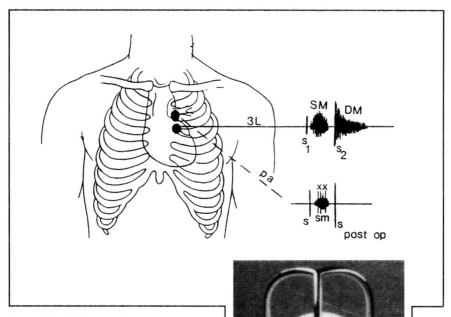

Figure 287: A 54-year-old woman with significant regurgitation. Because of her systolic murmur, some thought she had aortic stenosis; however, only regurgitation was actually present (documented at surgery). Before operation, systolic (SM) and diastolic murmurs (DM) were heard. A Starr-Edwards prosthetic valve replaced her damaged valve. Postoperatively, several systolic prosthetic valve sounds (xx) are heard over the pulmonic area. These sounds are produced by the prosthetic ball "jiggling" and striking the top of the cage. A midsystolic murmur (sm) also is present. These are normal findings in a patient with a Starr-Edwards valve. 3L = third left sternal border; pa = pulmonic area.

- **Clues to a Malfunctioning Valve — If a patient who has had a successful valve replacement for a condition such as mitral regurgitation, with significant improvement in symptoms, has return of the previous symptoms and signs of cardiac decompensation, always suspect a malfunctioning valve.**

A malfunctioning valve can be detected clinically or by procedures such as echocardiography.

An example — A patient who had a Starr-Edwards mitral valve prosthesis had excellent results following operation. After approximately one year, however, she had a return of symptoms of cardiac decompensation. On auscultation, the opening sound of the valve was abnormal. Instead of occurring at an interval after the second heart sound (like a third heart sound or the opening snap of mitral stenosis), it occurred

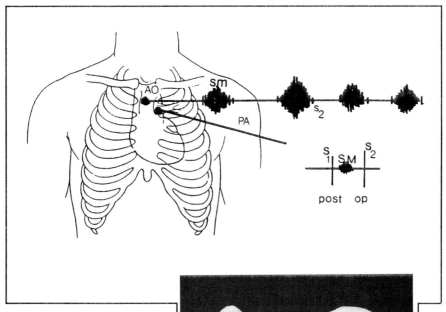

Figure 288: A 73-year-old man with severe aortic stenosis and advanced heart failure. He was incapacitated. A loud, long, harsh aortic systolic murmur (sm) was present. The second heart sound (S_2) is faint. Atrial fibrillation is also present. Note that, after a pause with atrial fibrillation, the murmur increases in intensity (second beat, top sketch). At surgery, a porcine valve replaced his stenotic one. A faint grade 2 to 3 systolic murmur is heard (SM) (bottom sketch, above), which is a normal finding for this valve. AO = aortic area; PA = pulmonic area; S_1 = first heart sound; S_2 = second heart sound.

much earlier in diastole, resembling a split second sound, and was heard over the mitral area. This meant that, in early diastole, the ball of the valve was not moving the entire distance of the enclosed cage, thereby causing the sound to occur earlier. That was a clue to malfunction of the valve.

Malfunction of a prosthetic heart valve can be caused by a number of things such as a clot in the cage or variance of the ball poppet due to cholesterol deposits or fracture. In the aforementioned patient, the problem was ball variance and the first valve was replaced with a new model Starr-Edwards valve. Her symptoms disappeared.

● **Diastolic Murmur in a Patient with a Prosthetic Valve — If a patient has a prosthetic valve inserted in the aortic position and an aortic diastolic murmur appears, suspect malfunction of the valve.**

Occasionally, the diastolic murmur may be of a faint degree, such as Grade 1 or Grade 2, and persists unchanged. In such a case, treatment may not be necessary. Very careful follow-up, of course, is necessary to make sure that the leak is not progressing. The occurrence of a significant leak that can be detected clinically is an indication for surgical correction.

Rheumatic Fever

- **Fifty percent of patients who have documented rheumatic fever do not develop a rheumatic heart. On the other hand, only 50% of those with mitral stenosis, which is a known complication of rheumatic fever, give a history of having had rheumatic fever (Figure 289).**

    This "50% rule" is an easy way to remember both of these observations.

- **There is a so-called rheumatic triad — rheumatic fever, mitral stenosis, atrial fibrillation. When two of these are present, the other will also be evident or probably will be forthcoming.**

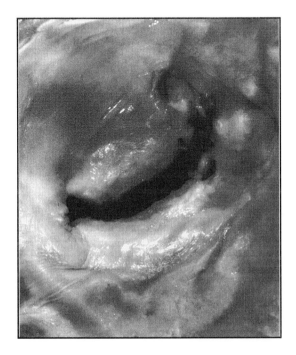

Figure 289: Mitral stenosis due to rheumatic fever. However only about 50% of these patients provide a known history of rheumatic fever.

For example, if a patient has mitral stenosis and a history of rheumatic fever, even though there is normal sinus rhythm at the time of your examination, it is likely that atrial fibrillation will develop in the future.

Is rheumatic fever having a resurgence? Recently, a significant number of new cases of rheumatic fever have been reported, so we should be aware of this and be on the lookout for them.

● **Rheumatic fever is most likely to affect both the aortic and mitral valves (Figure 290). Women are most likely to have more serious involvement of the mitral valve; in men it is the opposite; they have predominantly aortic valve involvement.**

Although most patients with rheumatic heart disease have lesions in both valves, occasionally there are exceptions; some patients have only mitral stenosis, even an advanced degree, without concomitant aortic valve involvement.

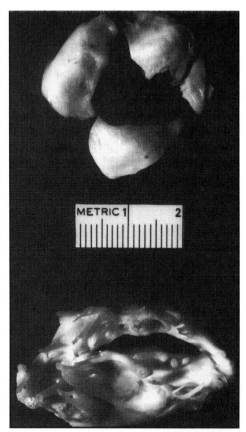

Figure 290: Rheumatic Heart Disease with aortic regurgitation (bottom) and mitral stenosis (top). Rheumatic hearts usually have *two* valves affected.

- **Carey-Coombs Diastolic Murmur** — The Carey-Coombs murmur is a diastolic murmur that can occur in patients who have acute rheumatic fever (Figure 291).

There is not much mention of this murmur these days, since rheumatic fever is uncommon, but in the past it was commonly noted and discussed. Rather than due to aortic regurgitation or mitral valve pathology, the most likely mechanism of this sound was a normal third heart sound having after vibrations of a low frequency rumble-type, plus low frequency vibrations that can occur with atrial contraction (S_4 or atrial sound). In a patient with a prolonged P-R interval due to first degree block, which can occur in acute rheumatic fever, the atrial contraction is in close proximity to the normal third heart sound. The combination of these two filling sounds with after vibrations can produce a rumble. Also, with the increase in heart rate that frequently occurs with rheumatic fever, diastole is shortened, causing two filling sounds, each with rumble vibrations occurring close together and producing the so-called Carey-Coombs murmur.

This is the same kind of diastolic rumble that occurs with dilated cardiomy-opathy. Thus the latter has been erroneously diagnosed as rheumatic mitral stenosis.

- **Aortic regurgitation occurring with acute rheumatic fever.**

I have personally observed patients who develop aortic regurgitation, even of a significant degree, with their first episode of acute rheumatic fever. Others have stated that this does not occur.

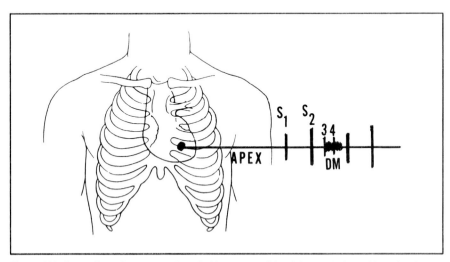

Figure 291: Carey-Coombs murmur heard with acute carditis of rheumatic fever: Note diastolic rumbling murmur (DM), probably the result of a third sound with low frequency after-vibrations in close proximity to an atrial (S_4) sound also having low frequency after-vibrations. The third and fourth sounds are close because of a prolonged P-R interval on the ECG plus a shortening of diastole due to an increased heart rate with the carditis.

- **Erythema Marginatum** — Erythema marginatum is a poorly recognized skin manifestation of rheumatic fever. The finding of slightly raised skin lesions, salmon-pinkish in color with scalloped edges, is an immediate clue as to the presence of rheumatic fever (Figure 292).

This skin eruption is more likely to occur on the front and back of the trunk — chest, abdomen and back, but can also occur on the arms and legs. Rubbing the area can help to bring out the lesions.

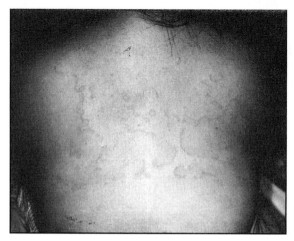

Figure 292: Erythema Marginatum — Very specific for active rheumatic fever.

Ventricular Septal Defect

- **Ventricular septal defect represents a common congenital heart lesion encountered in infants and children.**

- **A good proportion of small ventricular septal defects will close spontaneously with age.**

   A ventricular septal defect that is almost closed may not have the characteristic holosystolic (pansystolic) murmur. Instead, it may be a faint systolic murmur (Grade 1 to 3 in intensity) and occur in the first third of systole.

- **In the adult population, congenital aortic bicuspid valve is second to mitral valve prolapse as the most commonly encountered congenital lesion.**

- **Ventricular septal defects are classified as small, medium, and large. A majority of the small ventricular septal defects close during the first several years of life and some of the moderate sized ones may show some degree of closure, without actually doing so completely.**

- **Size of Defect** — **A small ventricular septal defect may produce no symptoms and the patient can lead a normal life. As mentioned, some close spontaneously.**

   Surgical closure is not often necessary. Prognosis is excellent. Infective endocarditis is a danger, however, so antibiotic prophylaxis is necessary before these patients have dental work, surgery or gastrointestinal or genitourinary instrumentation. Recommendations from the American Heart Association appear on page 83.

   One of our cardiac greats, a friend and colleague, the late Helen Taussig (Figure 293) of the Blalock-Taussig ("blue-baby") operation fame, provided the following cardiac pearl:

- **Operations on children should preferably be done before the age of six, since later in life they often do not have any memory of the operation.**

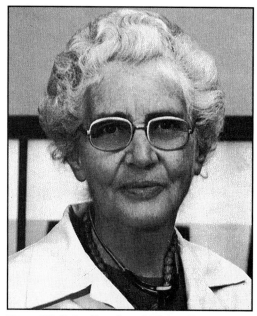

Figure 293: Helen Taussig — Of Blalock-Taussig ("blue baby") operation fame for Tetralogy of Fallot.

On the other hand, to operate after this age means taking the child out of school and now the operation can be a psychologically traumatic event which can affect the child in later life.

- **A holosystolic (pansystolic) murmur, Grade 3 to 4, is heard along the mid and lower left sternal border and apex. Since it is holosystolic (pansystolic), the differential diagnosis can be between ventricular septal defect, mitral regurgitation and tricuspid regurgitation.**

In a young patient (teenager and child), ventricular septal defect is the most common; however, if the patient is aged 30 to 40, do not diagnose ventricular septal defect as the first choice since it is very likely to be wrong and mitral regurgitation to be correct. Of course, ventricular septal defect is diagnosed in middle age and older, but mitral regurgitation due to mitral valve prolapse (floppy valve, rupture of chorda tendinea) is by far the most likely possibility. The ventricular septal defects of childhood may close spontaneously or be closed by surgery.

- **Third Heart Sound** — Helpful in the differentiation between ventricular septal defect and mitral regurgitation is the presence of a third heart sound heard at the lower left sternal border and apex. This is commonly found with mitral regurgitation but not with ventricular septal defect (unless the patient is in the younger age group where a normal physiological third heart sound is so prevalent).

- The holosystolic murmur detected along the lower left sternal border and apex brings up the differentiation between mitral regurgitation and ventricular septal defect. If it is a loud systolic murmur and accompanied by a palpable thrill, the ventricular septal defect thrill is along the left sternal border, whereas the mitral regurgitation thrill is at the apex.

If we examine 100 patients having uncomplicated ventricular septal defects, they will have a characteristic holosystolic murmur that peaks in midsystole. They may have a wider splitting of the second heart sound (Figure 294) presumably due to the simultaneous ejection of the left ventricular contents with systole, one going to the right side of the heart through the defect and the other to the aorta. Therefore, there is

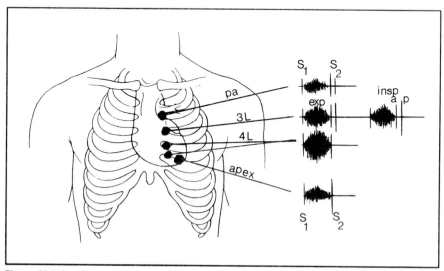

Figure 294: Another young woman with congenital ventricular defect. The holosystolic murmur is transmitted over the precordium, but is loudest at the fourth left sternal border (4L). The second sound is widely split (a-p) on inspiration and does not become single with expiration.

an earlier closure of the aortic component of the second heart sound. With mild to moderate degrees of ventricular septal defect, the second heart sound may be closely split or single on expiration, and widening with inspiration, as occurs normally. However, with more advanced and larger defects, there may be wider splitting both with expiration and inspiration; the split may widen slightly with inspiration but not return to single or closely split with expiration.

With the development of pulmonary hypertension producing the Eisenmenger type of ventricular septal defect, the pulmonic component (P_2) of the second heart sound becomes accentuated and the splitting is close (Figure 295). It generally does not become single, as some authors have described; instead of a single sound, one can detect a very narrow splitting of the second sound, widening slightly with inspiration.

With severe forms of pulmonary hypertension associated with ventricular septal defect there may be an ejection sound in the first part of systole and the former holosystolic murmur may now be a short murmur in the early to mid-portion of systole (Figure 296). In some patients with this advanced degree of pulmonary hypertension

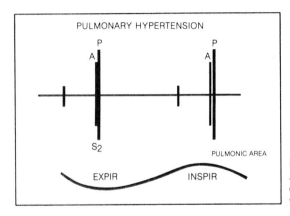

Figure 295: Pulmonary Hypertension — Accentuated, closely split second heart sound (S_2), due to loud pulmonic component (P_2), widens slightly with inspiration.

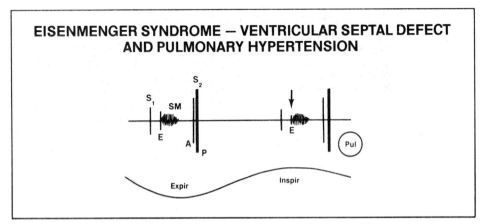

Figure 296: Accentuated, closely split second sound (A-P) widening slightly with inspiration. The ejection sound (E) decreases with inspiration and it's accompanied by a short early to midsystolic murmur (SM).

322

there can be a pulmonary diastolic regurgitation murmur that tapers off with high frequency components immediately following the second heart sound (Figure 297). The loud closure of P_2 can often be palpated. Sometimes the ejection sound can also be felt. A right ventricular impulse is usually present if searched for.

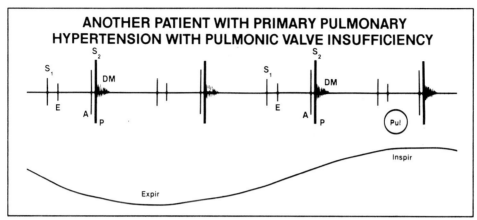

Figure 297: Accentuated, closely split second sound (A-P) which widens slightly with inspiration. The ejection sound (E) is unchanged by respiration. You will also hear a faint, short, early, blowing diastolic murmur (DM).

- **Can one distinguish the diastolic murmur of aortic regurgitation from that of hypertensive pulmonary regurgitation (Figure 298)? Yes. The aortic regurgitation murmur is accompanied by the palpation of a "quick rise or flip" (collapsing) type of peripheral arterial pulse, whereas the pulmonary regurgitation murmur is not.**

One may hear some components of the aortic regurgitation over the aortic area and transmitted to the apex. The pulmonary regurgitation would not likely be heard over the aortic area and is more localized along the left sternal border without transmission to the apex. On palpation of the precordium a left ventricular impulse consistent with aortic regurgitation would be felt at the apex. A right ventricular impulse of right ventricular hypertrophy would be felt at the lower left sternal border consistent with the hypertensive pulmonary regurgitation murmur.

Electrocardiogram and cardiac x-ray would, of course, show left ventricular hypertrophy with the aortic regurgitation and right hypertrophy, with the pathology causing pulmonary regurgitation.

Perforation of the Interventricular Septum

The differential is between that of a perforation of the interventricular septum and mitral valve pathology, including rupture of a papillary muscle. Some observers have stated that it is difficult to distinguish between these two conditions. However, there are cardiac pearls that can make this differentiation:

- The murmur of ventricular septal defect is usually best heard along the lower left sternal border, although there is radiation of this murmur to the apex (Figure 299). The murmur can be loud and heard in both places; however, if one carefully inches the stethoscope from the lower left sternal border to the apex, the murmur is loudest along the lower left sternal border area. The papillary muscle rupture is more likely to have the murmur loudest at the apex, with radiation laterally to the left axillary lines. Be sure to carefully search for a palpable thrill, for this may clinch the diagnosis. A palpable systolic thrill along the left sternal border is characteristic of septal perforation, whereas with

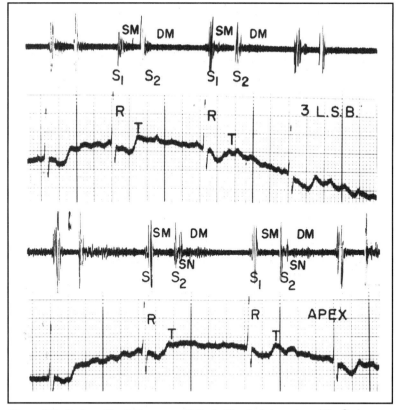

Figure 298: Graham-Steell Murmur — Patient with mitral stenosis and the Graham Steell murmur (DM) of pulmonic valve regurgitation (upper tracing). Note loud first sound (S$_1$), loud second sound (S$_2$), opening snap (S$_N$) and diastolic rumble (DM) (lower tracing).

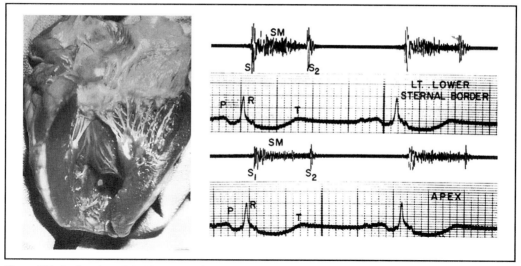

Figure 299: Perforation of the Ventricular Septum with myocardial infarction (left). The systolic murmur (SM) of ventricular septal defect is usually louder along the lower left sternal border (upper tracing) than at the apex (lower tracing) (right).

papillary muscle rupture the palpable systolic thrill is more likely localized over the apical area.

One physician may say that a systolic thrill is felt over the left sternal border, whereas another will state that a thrill is not felt. The explanation of this difference of observation is another cardiac pearl:

- **If one uses the tips of the fingers and strokes the inside of the opposite hand, moving from the tips of the fingers down to the wrist, it becomes evident that the most sensitive area is at the palm of the hand just at the junction of the fingers (Figure 300). Try this on both hands, since occasionally the area is even more sensitive on one hand as compared with the other.**

- **The physician who felt the palpable thrill used the palm of the hand in searching for the thrill, whereas the other physician used the tips of the fingers of the palpating hand and did not detect it. This explains the difference. Therefore, be sure to use the palm of the hand at the junction of the fingers when searching for a palpable thrill.**

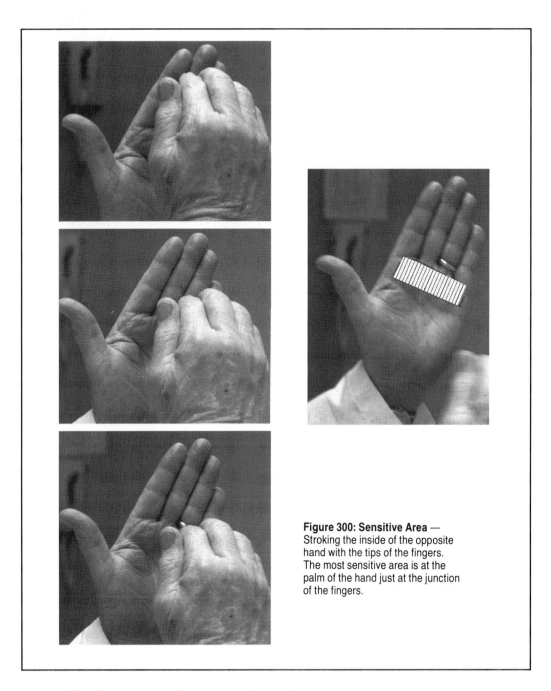

Figure 300: Sensitive Area —
Stroking the inside of the opposite
hand with the tips of the fingers.
The most sensitive area is at the
palm of the hand just at the junction
of the fingers.

The diagnosis can be accurately made at the bedside and fortunately today, these patients can often be salvaged by surgical correction. (It was not too many years ago that most died.)

- **The acute septal perforation associated with acute myocardial infarction represents a very serious complication, and early diagnosis and treatment is imperative, and can be life saving. A patient in the coronary care unit who has an acute myocardial infarction may have the sudden onset of pulmonary edema, shortness of breath, and chest pain. A loud systolic murmur, usually grade 4 or above, is heard along the left sternal border, and also can be heard at the apex. Pulsus alternans is present, with alternation of the second sound and alternation of the systolic murmur; a ventricular diastolic gallop is present in addition to an atrial (S_4) diastolic gallop. There is generally wider splitting of the second heart sound that may not become single with expiration.**

Uncommonly, the systolic murmur of septal perforation with acute myocardial infarction can be louder over the mitral area than along the left sternal border. A patient with this condition recently evaluated in the intensive care unit of St. Joseph's Hospital, Ann Arbor, Michigan, clearly had the louder murmur at the apex, although it was well heard over the lower left sternal border. A palpable systolic thrill was noted at the fourth left sternal border by two physicians and not over the mitral area.

The echocardiogram revealed a definite perforation at the lower part of the septum which probably explains the exception of the louder murmur over the mitral area. The cardiac pearl of diagnosis, however, was the low location of the perforation of the septum. The patient was obviously acutely ill, had cold clammy hands, extremities and body surface. She had Cheyne-Stokes respiration, faint thready arterial pulses, with pulsus alternans, alteration of the second sound and both ventricular (S_3) and atrial (S_4) gallops. She was promptly moved to the operating room for closure of her septal defect, which would be life saving. (Appreciation is expressed to Drs. Bruce Genovese and Ron Vanden Belt for allowing me to examine this patient and supplying details concerning her diagnostic workup which confirmed the clinical diagnosis of this condition.)

From a clinical standpoint, perforation of the intraventricular septum is much more common than that of papillary muscle rupture occurring with acute myocardial infarction. A cardiac pathologist I know states that he finds the papillary muscle rupture just about as common as the perforation of the intraventricular septum. This discrepancy in observation is probably related to the fact that as a pathologist he is not seeing those patients who survive the intraventricular septal perforations because of the excellent cardiac surgery to salvage them. Surgical correction of this dire complication represents another reversible form of heart disease.

On the other hand, the pathologist does examine the patients with papillary muscle rupture because death is more common. His observations of his own material are correct, but biased.

A few patients with the complication of perforation of the intraventricular septum with acute myocardial infarction may survive without surgery. Presumably this is possible because the perforation was of a smaller size, not causing the rapid fatal downhill course so characteristic of this complication of myocardial infarction. A few patients have been personally evaluated who had documented septal perforation but would not accept surgical correction. One such patient was a woman in her 60's who allowed cardiac catheterization but would not consider surgical correction. She remained in chronic cardiac decompensation and was presented in many teaching conferences. She subsequently died approximately four or five years following her myocardial infarction.

- **Helpful in the differentiation of the murmur of mitral regurgitation versus that of ventricular septal defect is the careful pinpointing of the location where the murmur is loudest. With ventricular septal defect it is best heard from the mid to the lower left sternal border and with mitral regurgitation it is best heard at the apex and with frequent radiation laterally to the midaxillary line, posterior axillary line and even to the posterior lung base (Figures 299 and 301).**

- **Windsock Sound — A ventricular septal defect that closes spontaneously may produce a sound in early systole, at the timing of an ejection sound. It is due to the bulging of the membranous closed or nearly closed defect, producing a sound analogous to a windsock that is distended, as seen at an airport (Figure 302).**

This sound occurs in early systole. It may be heard only (or better) with inspiration, not on expiration. This has been documented with angiograms showing the movement of this portion of the ventricular septum. This could also occur with a very small defect not completely closed.

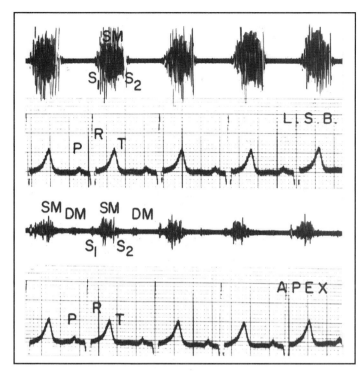

Figure 301: Patient with a Ventricular Septal Defect — Note systolic murmur (SM) peaking in midsystole; the murmur is louder along the lower left sternal border than at the apex.

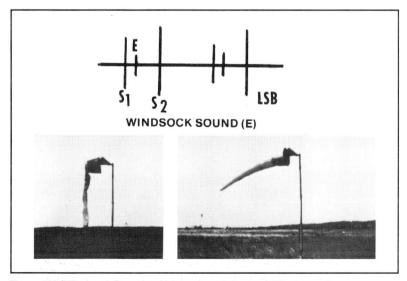

WINDSOCK SOUND (E)

Figure 302: Windsock Sound — Note early systolic sound (E) of a small closed (or nearly closed) ventricular septal defect. This has been aptly described as a "windsock" sound. Note "limp" windsock taken in an airport when there is no wind (bottom left) and when inflated and distended by the wind (bottom right).

Miscellaneous

It is wise to screen carefully for evidence of cardiac decompensation in patients who are to have surgery. As discussed previously (page 1) the detection of pulsus alternans, alternation of the intensity of the second sound and murmurs provides clues. If present and not diagnosed previously, then treatment can be instituted and the surgery can be delayed for several days. This is especially apropos for elderly patients with known or unknown cardiac decompensation. Taking extra days to make sure there is optimal medical control of the problem can be prophylactic against complications with surgery. For example, many patients are retaining extra edema fluid which can be removed with a mild diuretic. A word of caution, however, regarding a diuretic and loss of a significant amount of fluid. I recall reports of patients in the past who had a stroke coincident with the surgery; dehydration with the diuretic was thought to be a contributing factor. Therefore delay surgery for several days.

- **An electrocardiogram pre and postoperatively should be routine, as a myocardial infarction can occur during surgery and be "silent" because of the anesthesia.**

Pulmonary Hypertension

- **Clues on Physical Examination** — Signs of pulmonary hypertension include: A right ventricular lifting impulse along the lower left sternal border; a palpable pulmonic valve closure; possibly an A-wave detected on examination of the jugular venous pulse in the neck.

    On auscultation there may be a loud closely split second heart sound (Figure 303) (which might even be suspected on palpation), an ejection sound in early systole that becomes fainter on inspiration might be present, and with more advanced degrees of pulmonary hypertension, an atrial (S_4) gallop might be heard in presystole. If a systolic murmur is present it usually occurs in early to mid systole and is Grade 1 to 3 in intensity. In some patients an early, blowing, pulmonic diastolic murmur may be detected following the accentuated pulmonary component of the second heart sound.

- **Eisenmenger Syndrome** — The Eisenmenger syndrome is a specific sign of pulmonary hypertension that may be due to either ventricular septal defect, atrial septal defect, or patent ductus arteriosus.

    The second heart sound becomes accentuated, can be palpated over the pulmonic area, and becomes closely split. The second heart sound is loud due to the increased intensity of the pulmonary valve closure. Some observers have stated that the second heart sound becomes single with advanced degrees of pulmonary hypertension. However if one listens carefully, what at first may appear to be a single sound has a definite, albeit narrow, split. My personal observation has been that the splitting of the second heart sound is more pronounced in patients with the Eisenmenger syndrome due to atrial septal defect than in those with ventricular septal defect or patent ductus.

- **Syncope Due to Primary Pulmonary Hypertension** — Any time a young woman has episodes of syncope always think of primary pulmonary hypertension.

This is most common in teenaged girls or women in their 20's or 30's. The syncope generally occurs with some degree of exertion, though not necessarily strenuous. No one seems to know why this affects women more than men.

I recall two patients. The first was a young woman about 20 years of age who had syncope on even moderate exertion, such as carrying a bag of groceries up a slight incline. Another, a man in his 20's, was a delivery man. He had syncopal episodes when lifting or carrying even more moderate sized packages. Both had primary pulmonary hypertension.

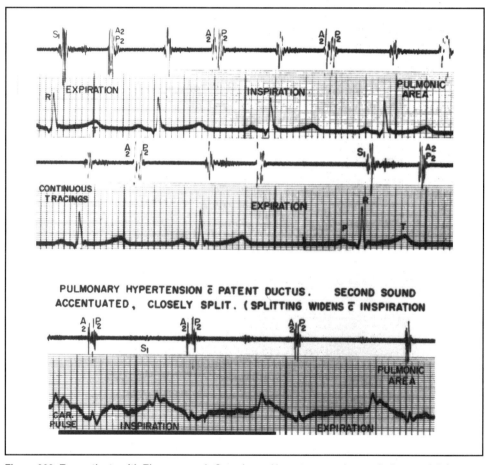

Figure 303: Two patients with Eisenmenger's Complex — Upper two sounds: ventricular septal defect with pulmonary hypertension. Note closely split accentuated second sound ($A_2 P_2$) which widens on inspiration. Lowest panel: patent ductus. The loud second sound ($A_2 P_2$) is closely split with expiration and widens on inspiration.

- **Congenital Pulmonary Valve Regurgitation** — The diastolic murmur due to a congenital pulmonary valve regurgitation occurs with a low pressure circuit as contrasted to the high pressure pulmonary hypertensive diastolic murmur. The hypertensive diastolic *high frequency* murmur immediately "tails off" the loud pulmonic component of the closely split second sound. The murmur of congenital pulmonary valve regurgitation usually occurs after a pause following closure of the second sound and may have rumble-like, low frequency components; this murmur increases coincidentally with inspiration (Figures 304 and 305).

Occasionally congenital pulmonary valve regurgitation occurs closely after the pulmonic valve closure, but usually there is a definite pause and this pause before the murmur occurs is a cardiac pearl in diagnosis of this condition. The murmur often increases with inspiration. The outlook is excellent for the great majority of patients with congenital pulmonary valve regurgitation; they are able to tolerate this type of leak without difficulty.

A murmur due to pulmonary regurgitation is frequently heard after repair of a Tetralogy of Fallot. This also may occur following a pause after the second sound and also may increase in intensity on inspiration. As a rule, this murmur, too, is well tolerated by the patient, causing no symptoms.

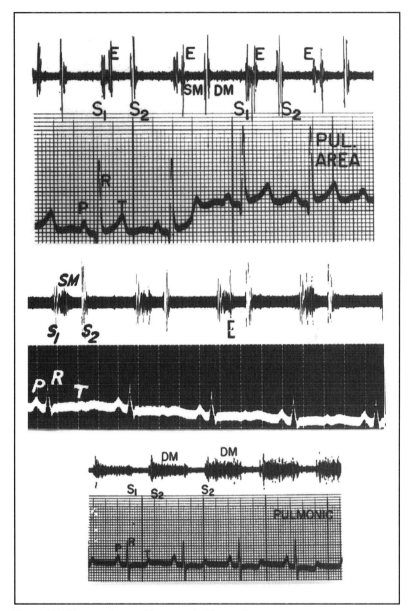

Figure 304: Three patients with congenital heart disease and pulmonary hypertension. Top tracing: Note prominent second sound (S_2) and ejection sound (E); and faint systolic (SM) and diastolic (DM) murmurs. Middle tracing: Ventricular septal defect. Note early systolic murmur (SM) and ejection sound (E), and loud S_2. Bottom panel: Another patient with patent ductus and pulmonary hypertension — A loud, high frequency diastolic murmur (DM) is heard. It simulated a loud aortic diastolic murmur.

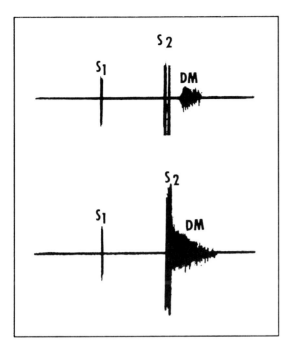

Figure 305: Two types of pulmonary regurgitation.
Top: Low pressure pulmonary regurgitation. The diastolic
murmur (DM) may be heard after a pause following the
second sound (S₂). The murmur can increase coincident
with inspiration. No pulmonary hypertension is present.
Bottom: High pressure pulmonary regurgitation.
Pulmonary hypertension is present. Note diastolic
murmur "tails off" the loud second sound.

Tricuspid Stenosis

- **What may be a new auscultatory finding** (at least for me): **If a rheumatic heart has a diastolic rumble with presystolic accentuation best heard over the tricuspid area (lower left sternal border) increasing with inspiration, and there is a *normal or only slightly accentuated first heart sound*, plus a *faint (often overlooked) opening snap of the mitral valve,* suspect the presence of predominant tricuspid stenosis along with mild to moderate mitral valve stenosis.**

      This murmur of the tricuspid stenosis may be best heard over the lower left sternal border, but may also be detected at the apex; clues as to the predominance of tricuspid stenosis over mitral stenosis are (Figure 306): the faint opening snap, a first sound not particularly accentuated, plus the diastolic rumble with presystolic accentuation heard best over the tricuspid area and strikingly increasing coincident with inspiration. This is the diastolic rumble of tricuspid stenosis.

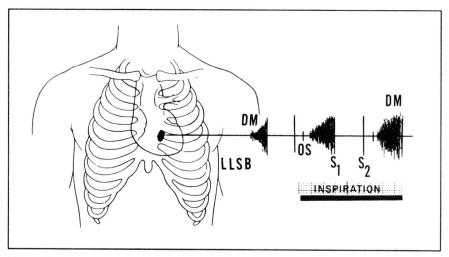

Figure 306: Patient with predominant tricuspid stenosis and mild mitral stenosis. Note first sound (S₁) is not accentuated. The opening snap (OS) is faint. The diastolic rumble (DM) greatly increases in intensity with inspiration.

Remember, when both rheumatic mitral and tricuspid stenosis coexist, and mitral stenosis is the dominant lesion (Figure 307), the first heart sound is loud, as is the second sound; the opening snap is easily heard over the tricuspid area, as is the diastolic rumble, often with presystolic accentuation and not becoming louder with inspiration.

When the rhythm is regular, the "tight" mitral stenosis produces a long diastolic rumble beginning after the opening snap, and continuing throughout diastole, and with presystolic accentuation. It is best heard over the point of maximal impulse of the left ventricle with the patient turned to the left lateral position. On the other hand, the usual presystolic rumbling murmur of tricuspid stenosis is best heard over the lower left sternal border (tricuspid area). This characteristic murmur often does not crescendo up to the first heart sound (Figure 308). Instead there is a pause *after the murmur* (an auscultatory gap) and then the first sound is heard. The P-R interval on the ECG is often prolonged, which may contribute to the gap. The diastolic rumble can show a striking increase in intensity coincident with inspiration, which can also be associated with a prominent "A" wave in the jugular venous pulse.

- **Murmurs of Tricuspid Stenosis — The murmurs of tricuspid stenosis, most commonly heard in patients with rheumatic heart disease, have concomitant mitral stenosis and about 25% to 33% of these patients have concomitant aortic valve disease with stenosis and/or insufficiency.**

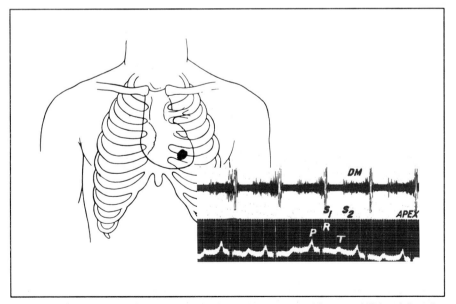

Figure 307: Patient with Predominant Mitral Stenosis — Note loud first sound (S_1) and diastolic rumble (DM) filling all of diastole.

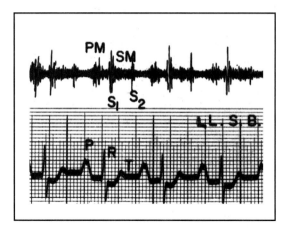

Figure 308: Murmur of Tricuspid Stenosis — The presystolic murmur (PM) dose not crescendo up to the first sound (S_1). Instead, there is a pause after the murmur probably contributed to by the prolonged P-R interval. LLSB = lower left sternal area (tricuspid area).

- **Tricuspid Regurgitation** — **The murmur of tricuspid regurgitation is best heard along the lower left sternal border. It is generally holosystolic (or pansystolic) and increases coincident with inspiration (Figures 309 and 310).**

   The earliest degrees of tricuspid regurgitation, such as may initially occur with infective endocarditis in a heroin addict, may be very subtle, a systolic murmur may be heard only with inspiration and can occur in early to mid-systole rather than be pansystolic. An atrial sound (S_4) may also be present and become more evident with inspiration (Figure 311). On the other end of the spectrum, the most wide open, patulous valves having the most advanced degrees of tricuspid regurgitation might not even show the presence of a murmur; if present, the murmur might not increase with inspiration.

- **Right Ventricular Infarction** — **Right ventricular infarction, although uncommon, does occur. It may be associated with significant tricuspid regurgitation.**

   A prominent V-wave as noted in the jugular venous pulse may increase with inspiration, also producing an increase in the tricuspid systolic murmur. The more advanced degrees of tricuspid regurgitation can even cause systolic movement of the ear lobes as well as a rightward lateral movement of the head coincident with systole. (This has been called the "no-no" sign as compared with the "yes-yes" sign of advanced aortic regurgitation which produces the "up and down" bobbing of the head).

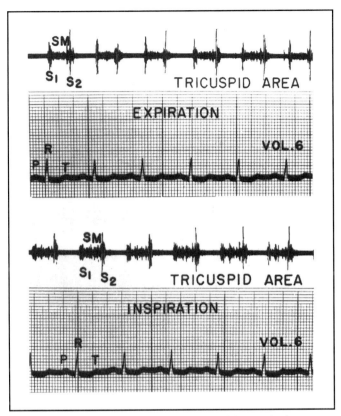

Figure 309: The pansystolic murmur of tricuspid regurgitation increases with inspiration.

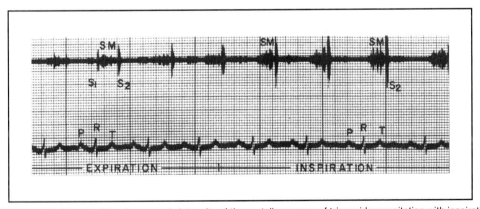

Figure 310: Note striking increase in intensity of the systolic murmur of tricuspid regurgitation with inspiration.

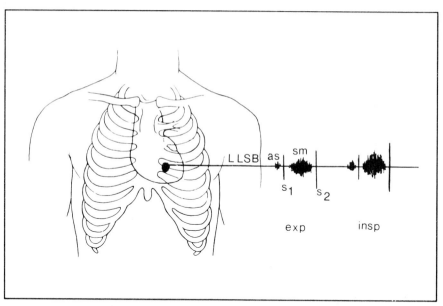

Figure 311: A heroin addict who has infective endocarditis on his tricuspid valve. An atrial systolic murmur (as) is heard in presystole and a systolic murmur (sm) is present, both becoming louder on inspiration. The heart sounds (S_1, S_2) also get louder with inspiration. Prominent "a" and "v" waves were noted in the right jugular venous pulse. LLSB = the right tricuspid area, the lower left sternal border.

Cardiopulmonary Resuscitation

I recently participated in a Cardiac Symposium and heard Dr. Gordon Ewy, Professor and Chief of Cardiology, University of Arizona College of Medicine, speak on cardiopulmonary resuscitation. He presented the following pertinent cardiac pearls:

"The optimal approach to cardiopulmonary resuscitation has changed somewhat over the last several years. Critical factors necessary for successful CPR include the following:

"In all arrests due to ventricular fibrillation, the critical step is defibrillation and if prompt, no other intervention is necessary. If defibrillation is delayed, usually because of the location of the cardiac arrest, then basic CPR techniques are necessary to slow the process of organ deterioration until defibrillation can be applied.

"Accordingly, in out-of-hospital cardiac arrest, one of the major determinants of survival is the time to onset of basic CPR and the time to defibrillation. Time to onset of basic CPR is shortened with the initiation of bystander CPR. If bystander CPR is initiated within four minutes and definitive therapy within eight minutes, 43% of patients with ventricular fibrillation survive to leave the hospital. If CPR is not initiated by a bystander and is not begun until the ambulance or paramedic arrive even when the units arrive within eight minutes, survival decreases to 27%. If definitive therapy is delayed by more than eight minutes, survival is rare.

"Because of these facts, efforts are being made to encourage bystander CPR."

- **Surveys indicate that many individuals are reluctant to perform bystander CPR because of the fear of infection from mouth-to-mouth ventilation.**

"Accordingly, we studied the feasibility of performing only chest compression during the first 12 minutes of CPR and found in our experimental model that when promptly initiated, **chest compression alone was as effective as basic CPR with both ventilation and chest compression.**

"The new guidelines have made one major change in basic CPR recommendations. Since early defibrillation is critical to survival, the bystander is to call 911 *first* before initiating CPR. This will help to decrease the delay in arrival of definitive therapy.

"Other attempts to improve early response have been the recommendation of chest thump for witnessed arrest, and the placement of automatic defibrillators in ambulances, in isolated areas, or in areas where large numbers of people susceptible to arrest congregate.

- **The technique of chest compression during CPR is important. It has now been demonstrated that cardiac compression is the mechanism of blood flow during closed chest CPR, and therefore forceful sternal compression at 100 compressions per minute (metronome guided when possible) are necessary.**

"The drug of choice in CPR is epinephrine. High dose epinephrine is not better than standard dose, and high dose is probably detrimental.

"Sodium bicarbonate is not necessary during the first 15 minutes of CPR and calcium carbonate is contraindicated except in rare situations where hypocalcemia is present. Isoproterenol is also contraindicated since the beneficial effect of epinephrine is its alpha adrenergic effect. Epinephrine works well when given with a beta blocker but not at all when given with an alpha blocker, leaving only its beta stimulating properties, like isoproterenol."

Dr. Ewy is one of our country's authorities on cardiopulmonary resuscitation. He also mentioned that there is now an apparatus available to perform the chest compression and it is effective. Apropos of this: Perhaps you read in the newspaper a report of successful CPR resulting from the use of a toilet plunger used for chest compression – good, quick thinking, which makes sense.

Cardiac Transplantation

Selection of Patients — As a result of the pioneering and continuing work of Dr. Norman Shumway of Stanford University, cardiac transplantation represents a major advance in treatment of end stage cardiac disease. It is performed throughout the world and at the present time the great majority of patients who receive a heart transplant are living at the end of one year.

Obviously, we must be conservative about advising this procedure. Within one recent year, I personally observed three patients who were advised to have cardiac transplantation and put on a waiting list. We advised all to take more time on conservative medical treatment before having the surgery. All had dilated cardiomyopathy, which can cover a spectrum from mild to severe. It is possible that some patients who are in an advanced stage of dilated cardiomyopathy can have some regression back to the moderate degrees of the spectrum and lead a comfortable life. Those in the mild degrees can reverse to normal if there is early recognition and early treatment (particularly physical rest). However, some with seemingly mild involvement initially can progress to moderate or severe degrees of the spectrum.(Fig. 128)

One patient, who had the type of cardiomyopathy seen during and after pregnancy, had apparently been advised that, if after several months there was no improvement in her advanced heart failure, it was unlikely that further conservative medical treatment would be helpful. However, the cardiac transplant was deferred and the patient was taken off the waiting list; one year later she is much improved, though still in the moderate degree of the spectrum; she has been able to return to work on a part time basis.

Another patient is now approximately one year later and continues to improve to a degree that it appears that the cardiac transplantation may not be necessary. The third patient is now three years after he followed advice to go the path of continued stricter medical treatment and he has shown a significant improvement, having returned to the daily work of his occupation. Of course, patients in the most severe degree of the spectrum cannot be reversed and cardiac transplantation can be lifesaving.

- **Cardiac Pearl: A basic, simple, but important aspect of medical treatment is *physical* rest. Of course, other medical treatments for heart failure must be employed concomitantly. Nevertheless, early suspicion, early diagnosis, and early treatment, specifically with physical rest can result in reversal of a course that would otherwise almost certainly be progressively downhill.**

Obviously, there are many more cardiac pearls that are not included in this book at the present time. However, in a subsequent edition, perhaps this can be done.

Thank you for reading these cardiac pearls, which I hope have been interesting and informative for you.

Tentative plans are currently under way to provide a supplement to this edition of Cardiac Pearls in the form of high fidelity cassette tape recordings of heart sounds from actual patients correlated with the written text.

Sincerely,

W. Proctor Harvey M.D.

W. Proctor Harvey

Acknowledgements

In preparation of this book, I would like to acknowledge, with sincere thanks, the contributions and support of many people:

My wife Irma and sons, Proctor Jr. and Blair.

My friends and colleagues with whom I have worked for several decades on a number of teaching and educational projects.

David and Anne Canfield

Georgetown faculty; residents and students who number in the thousands.

Special thanks to our Georgetown Cardiology Fellows, past and present, from whom I have learned much. I am proud of their dedication, excellence and G/T (give/take) ratio.

Bernard Salb, former Head of Photography at Georgetown, for his outstanding work over many years, which contributed significantly to this book.

Ruth Weinmann, super nurse and technician.

Georgetown secretaries: Jonnie Morrow and Mary McAuliffe

Melinda Decker, for her secretarial work

Mary Johnson Wright, for her design and mechanical preparation

Eda Levy, for proofreading

Jerry, a patient, for his encouragement and help

Bill Roberts, for teaching all of us cardiac pathology

Tony deLeon, for his friendship and continuing assistance over the years

Charles Hufnagel, pioneer cardiovascular surgeon

Appreciation for permission to reproduce the following figures:

      Figs. 127 and 208 – Bruce Waller

      Fig. 168 – Wide World Photo

      Fig. 169 – American Journal of Cardiology

      Fig. 148 – Dr. Bob Hall

      Fig. 220 – Dr. Helen Taussig

      Fig. 292 – Dr. Virginia Sulica

      Fig. 282 – Dr. William Baker

      Figs. 250 and 270 – Dr. Donald Knowlan

Many figures in this book, or portions of figures, are from the author's textbook, *Clinical Auscultation of the Heart,* W.B. Saunders Co., and are reproduced with permission. All phonocardiograms were taken solely by the author.

Some of the author's material has also been used with permission of Laennec Publishing Co., from *Clinical Auscultation of the Cardiovascular System,* by Harvey and Canfield and *Cardiovascular Evaluation of Athletes,* Waller and Harvey, editors.